SPORTS AND ATHLETICS PREPARATION, PERFORMANCE
AND PSYCHOLOGY

TRENDS IN HUMAN PERFORMANCE RESEARCH

SPORTS AND ATHLETICS PREPARATION, PERFORMANCE, AND PSYCHOLOGY

Additional books in this series can be found on Nova's website under the Series tab.

Additional E-books in this series can be found on Nova's website under the E-book tab.

SPORTS AND ATHLETICS PREPARATION, PERFORMANCE
AND PSYCHOLOGY

TRENDS IN HUMAN PERFORMANCE RESEARCH

MICHAEL J. DUNCAN
AND
MARK LYONS
EDITORS

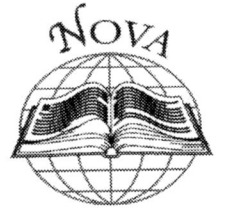

Nova Science Publishers, Inc.
New York

Copyright © 2010 by Nova Science Publishers, Inc.

All rights reserved. No part of this book may be reproduced, stored in a retrieval system or transmitted in any form or by any means: electronic, electrostatic, magnetic, tape, mechanical photocopying, recording or otherwise without the written permission of the Publisher.

For permission to use material from this book please contact us:
Telephone 631-231-7269; Fax 631-231-8175
Web Site: http://www.novapublishers.com

NOTICE TO THE READER

The Publisher has taken reasonable care in the preparation of this book, but makes no expressed or implied warranty of any kind and assumes no responsibility for any errors or omissions. No liability is assumed for incidental or consequential damages in connection with or arising out of information contained in this book. The Publisher shall not be liable for any special, consequential, or exemplary damages resulting, in whole or in part, from the readers' use of, or reliance upon, this material. Any parts of this book based on government reports are so indicated and copyright is claimed for those parts to the extent applicable to compilations of such works.

Independent verification should be sought for any data, advice or recommendations contained in this book. In addition, no responsibility is assumed by the publisher for any injury and/or damage to persons or property arising from any methods, products, instructions, ideas or otherwise contained in this publication.

This publication is designed to provide accurate and authoritative information with regard to the subject matter covered herein. It is sold with the clear understanding that the Publisher is not engaged in rendering legal or any other professional services. If legal or any other expert assistance is required, the services of a competent person should be sought. FROM A DECLARATION OF PARTICIPANTS JOINTLY ADOPTED BY A COMMITTEE OF THE AMERICAN BAR ASSOCIATION AND A COMMITTEE OF PUBLISHERS.

LIBRARY OF CONGRESS CATALOGING-IN-PUBLICATION DATA

Trends in research / Michael J. Duncan.
 p. cm.
 Includes index.
 ISBN 978-1-61668-591-1 (hardcover)
 1. Sports--Physiological aspects. I. Duncan, Michael J.
 RC1235.T725 2009
 613.7'1072--dc22

2010012258

Published by Nova Science Publishers, Inc. † *New York*

CONTENTS

Preface		vii
Chapter 1	Placebo Effects of Caffeine on Hockey Skill Performance	1
	Samantha Taylor and Michael J. Duncan	
Chapter 2	The Effect of Using Hiking Poles on O_2 Uptake, Heart Rate and Blood Lactate During Uphill Walking	9
	Joseph Moreton and Michael J. Duncan	
Chapter 3	Anthropometric Profiles of Elite Junior Ice-Hockey Players	17
	Joanne Hankey, Mark Lyons and Michael J. Duncan	
Chapter 4	The Impact of Caffeine Consumption on 1000-Metre Rowing Performance	23
	Michael J. Duncan	
Chapter 5	New Applications for Encouraging Fitness	35
	Dorota Groffik and Karel Frömel	
Chapter 6	Structural Analysis of Basic Leg Extensor Isometric F-T Curve Characteristics in Male Athletes in Different Sports Measured in Standing Position	53
	Milivoj Dopsaj, Miroljub Blagojevic, Nenad Koropanovski, and Goran Vuckovic	

Chapter 7	Acute Effects of Variable Resistance Exercise on Force and Power Characteristics During the Back Squat Exercise	71
	Philip H. Watkins and Gareth Richards	
Chapter 8	Sensorimotor Exercises in Sports Training and Rehabilitation	79
	Erika Zemková	
Chapter 9	Dietary Calcium – A Potential Ergogenic Aid?	119
	Rehana Jawadwala	
Chapter 10	Active Video Game Play – A Novel and Useful Exercise Modality?	139
	Mark Willems	
Chapter 11	Augmented Eccentric Loading: Theoretical and Practical Applications	151
	Philip H. Watkins	
Chapter 12	Predictors of Exercise Performance	167
	Ahmad Alkhatib	
Index		189

PREFACE

Achievements related to human performance have recently surpassed what was once thought possible. In part, these developments are due to greater understanding of the scientific factors that underpin performance in tasks related to all aspects of human movement. This has included advances in varied academic domains such as exercise physiology, nutrition, strength and conditioning, psychology, ergonomics and physical therapy. This book presents recent research in the field that provides a bridge between scientific knowledge and practitioners involved in the enhancement of human performance.

Short communication A presents data on psychological aspects of nutritional manipulation with an examination of the placebo effect of caffeine on sport specific skill performance. Short communication B provides the reader with an insight into the role of hiking poles of the physiological responses to uphill walking, thus illustrating how particular equipment may influence human exertional performance and short communication C identifies positional differences in the anthropometric profiles of junior ice-hockey players which has possible application to the development of sport specific training programmes and talent identification in ice-hockey.

A number of research articles are also presented which provide interesting practical applications and directions for future research. Chapter I identifies improvements in short term rowing performance as a result of caffeine intake and Chapter II investigates the physical activity patterns of children and the possible role that pedometers may have in enhancing young people's physical activity. Chapter III provides the reader with background on the structural properties in basic leg extensor function across male performers from various sports. Chapter IV follows on this theme by investigating the acute impact of using chain based loads on force and power during resistance exercise.

Several review articles are also presented which provide the reader with relevant, up-to-date information pertinent to a range of areas related to human performance. Chapter V supplies the reader with key information relating to the use of sensorimotor exercises that practitioners could use in both sport specific training and in rehabilitation from injury whilst chapter VI identifies the potential ergogenic properties of calcium, a nutrient that has previously been overlooked in the literature compared to other methods of dietary manipulation. Chapter VII provides an insightful overview of an emerging research area, active video games, as an alternative exercise modality compared to more traditional forms of exercise and physical activity. The focus of chapter VIII is the use of augmented eccentric loading in enhancing human strength and power. This chapter provides applied information that can be used by those working with both high level athletic groups as well as with the general population. In Chapter VIIII a review on predictors of exercise performance is provided. This focuses on issues such as lactate responses to exercise, lactate as a predictor of performance and the role of lactate in carbohydrate and fat utilization during exercise. This chapter has clear applicability to practitioners and coaches interested n enhancing aerobically based performance.

It is hoped that this text provides a broad and balanced overview of a range of topics relevant to individuals working within the field of human performance. Whilst this field is vast in terms of the disciplines it encompasses, the chapters in this book are drawn from a range of disciplines including exercise physiology, nutrition, physical activity, biomechanics, psychology and sports therapy and rehabilitation. Hopefully, the information presented here will prompt discussion, further research and stimulate further improvements in the scientific enhancement of human performance.

Michael J. Duncan and Mark Lyons

In: Trends in Human Performance Research
Editors: M. Duncan and M. Lyons

ISBN: 978-1-61668-591-1
© 2010 Nova Science Publishers, Inc.

Chapter 1

PLACEBO EFFECTS OF CAFFEINE ON HOCKEY SKILL PERFORMANCE

Samantha Taylor[1]* and Michael J. Duncan[2]
Nottingham Trent University, UK
Coventry University, UK

ABSTRACT

Recent research has indicated improved aerobic performance after caffeine consumption. However, few studies have examined placebo effects on skilled sports performance. The aim of this study was to examine the placebo effect of caffeine on motor skill performance. Following ethics approval and informed consent, 9 male and 7 female university hockey players (mean age = 21 ± 1.8 years) volunteered to participate. Participants completed a hockey skills test under 3 conditions: control, placebo and a caffeine condition. However, no caffeine was administered, instead a deceptive administration protocol was used and 300ml of an orange flavored drink was consumed 30 minutes prior to testing in both the placebo and caffeine conditions. During each condition, participants completed the Chapman Test protocol as a

---

* Please address all correspondence to: Michael J. Duncan,
Department of Biomolecular and Sports Science,
James Starley Building, Coventry University,
Coventry, United Kingdom
Email: michael.duncan@Coventry.ac.uk

measure of hockey ball handling ability and provided RPE indicators. Results indicated there were significant differences in stick handling ability across the three conditions (P = 0.001). Bonferroni post hoc tests indicated that performance was better in the perceived caffeine condition compared to the control condition (P= 0.01), and in the perceived caffeine condition compared to the perceived placebo condition (P = 0.024). Scores in the perceived placebo condition were also significantly better compared with the control condition (P=0.009). RPE scores were higher in the control condition compared to both the perceived caffeine (P =0.01) and perceived placebo conditions (P =0.01). The results suggest that when participants believed they had consumed caffeine, hockey skill improved in comparison to perceived placebo and control conditions.

Keywords: Chapman Test, Motor Skill, Performance.

INTRODUCTION

The positive impact of caffeine ingestion on endurance capacity, particularly prolonged and exhaustive exercise has been well-established (Graham, 2001). However, recent research has suggested that performance enhancement from caffeine may be a result of psychological factors rather than true physiological change (Beedie et al., 2006). The 'placebo effect' is often used to explain how a desired outcome occurs when an individual believes they have received a beneficial treatment, when in fact they have not. In such cases it is the participant's belief which has heralded the results (Foad et al., 2008; Beedie et al 2006).

Despite evidence that the placebo effect impacts on a range of variables, its influence related to sport and exercise performance has received limited attention (Foad et al., 2008). Some studies have suggested that placebo effects are associated with improved aerobic endurance (Beedie et al., 2006; Clark et al., 2000) and improved short term, high-intensity exercise (Duncan e al., 2009). Beedie et al. (2006) reported a 2.2% increase in mean power, above baseline, when cyclists thought they had consumed caffeine compared to a 1% increase when they thought they had consumed placebo during a 10km time trial. More recently, Duncan et al. (2009) reported placebo effects of caffeine during an acute bout of resistance exercise with participants completing significantly more repetitions to failure when they believed they had consumed caffeine compared to the perceived placebo condition.

This topic is important as nutritional supplementation, including caffeine use, is widely employed in both recreational and competitive sport and exercise settings and although research related to placebo effects in sport is emerging, few studies have examined placebo effects on skilled sports performance (Fillmore and Vogel-Sprott, 1992). Therefore, the aim of this study was to examine the placebo effect of caffeine on skilled sports performance.

METHOD

Participants

Following ethics approval and informed consent, 9 male and 7 female university hockey players (mean age ± S.D. = 21 ± 1.8 years) volunteered to participate in this study. The participants were informed that they were participating in a study examining the effect of caffeine on hockey performance where they would be required to consume 2 solutions, one containing 5mg kg^{-1} of caffeine and one containing a placebo.

Procedure

Each participant was required to attend four testing sessions, one familiarization and 3 experimental conditions. In the familiarization session, participants completed 20 trials of the Chapman Hockey skills test to ensure equity of learning prior to the experimental trials.

Experimental conditions were presented in a randomised order and separated by 24-72 hours. One condition was used as a control trial and involved no consumption of any substance. In the other 2 trials participants were informed that they would consume 5mg kg^{-1} of caffeine or a placebo diluted into a solution on a randomly assigned double-blind basis. However, a deceptive administration protocol was employed whereby participants only consumed 300ml of an artificially sweetened drink 60 minutes before each exercise trial. During each condition, participants completed a 5 minute submaximal warm-up and then completed the Chapman Hockey Test protocol (Chapman, 1982 cited in Strand, and Wilson, 1993). The Chapman protocol is a well validated measure of hockey stick handling ability where participants are required to dribble a hockey ball into the centre of the target area through one third of a peripheral circle and dribble the ball out of an alternative circle segment as many times as possible in 30 seconds with higher scores reflecting greater stick handling ability.

In addition, on completion of each hockey test, participants were asked to rate his perception of exertion using the Borg 6-20 RPE Scale (Borg, 1970) in order to assess the perceptual response to each condition.

Statistical Analysis

Any changes in stick handling ability and RPE were examined using 3-way repeated measures, analysis of variance (ANOVA). Post hoc analysis using Bonferroni adjustments were performed where any significant interactions and main effects were found. A P value of 0.05 was used to establish statistical significance and the Statistical Package for Social Sciences (SPSS, Inc, Chicago, Ill) Version 17.0 was used for all analyses.

RESULTS

Results indicated there were significant differences in stick handling ability across the three conditions ($F_{2, 30} = 12.379$, $P = 0.001$). Bonferroni post hoc tests indicated that performance was better in the perceived caffeine condition compared to the control condition (Mean Diff = 5.063, P= 0.01), and in the perceived caffeine condition compared to the perceived placebo condition (Mean Diff = 2.06, P = 0.024). Scores in the perceived placebo condition were also significantly better compared with the control (Mean Diff = 3.000, P=0.009). Mean ± S.D. of scores on the Chapman test across conditions are presented in Figure 1.

With regard to RPE, results also indicated significant differences across conditions ($F_{2, 30} = 11.503$, $P = 0.01$) with higher RPE scores in the control condition compared to both the perceived caffeine (Mean diff = 3.125, P = 0.01) and perceived placebo conditions (Mean diff = 3.125, P =0.01). There was no significant difference in RPE scores between the perceived caffeine and perceived placebo conditions (P > 0.05). Mean ± S.D. of RPE was 17.1 ± 1.3, 14.1 ± 3.2 and 14 ± 1.7 for control, perceived placebo and perceived caffeine conditions respectively.

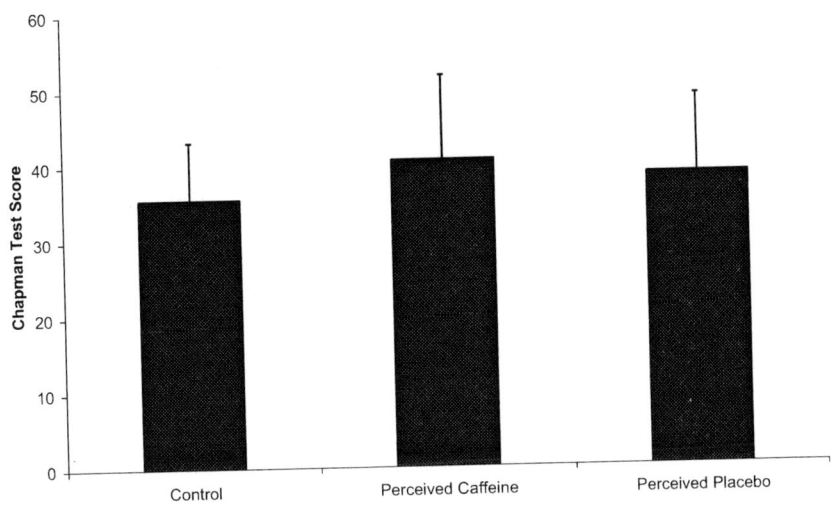

Figure 1. Mean ± S.D. of scores on the Chapman Hockey test across conditions.

DISCUSSION

The results of this study raise some interesting issues. Principally, when individuals in this study consumed a substance which they believed to be caffeine they performed better on a test of hockey stick handling ability compared to when they had consumed a substance they believed to be placebo. These results support the findings of prior studies that have examined placebo effects during both aerobic and resistance exercise (Beedie et al., 2006; Duncan et al., 2009). These results also agree with the only other study that has examined placebo effects on motor skill performance (Fillmore and Vogel-Sprott, 1992). The results of this study in regard to RPE also concur with other studies that reported dampened RPE during exercise when caffeine was consumed compared to placebo (Docherty and Smith, 2005). However, it is also possible that decreased RPE during the perceived placebo condition could be as a result of a placebo effect.

Possible placebo effect mechanisms to explain increases in performance as a result of consuming what they believe to be a particular substance have been proposed (Beedie et al., 2006) but it is not known whether the placebo effect is manifest as a direct effect on performance or whether because the participant becomes more aware in searching for caffeine related symptoms it leads to changes in performance strategy. As no direct measure of physiological strain was assessed in the current study, this could be considered a limitation and should be addressed in future research.

The placebo effect may not be the only explanation for the findings of the current study. This effect relies on a relationship between beliefs and performance. It may be in the current study that the differences between conditions were as a result of low a priori expectations of performance in the perceived placebo condition or because of the motivational climate fostered by the situation. If a performer had low expectations in the condition that they believed was the placebo condition any statistical difference in performance between the perceived caffeine and perceived placebo trials may have been magnified. Motivational climate was not considered in the current study and future research is warranted which takes into account issues such as personality, motivational climate and responsiveness when examining placebo effects. This study employed university standard Hockey players. It may also be interesting for practitioners to examine whether the placebo effect on sport-specific motor skills are manifest across levels of expertise within a given sport.

Finally, use of a deceptive administration protocol as has been used in the current study, is predicated on the fact that participants are told that they will be taking a particular substance and so the experimental data is not truly blind. Recent research by Foad et al. (2008) has used the double disassociation design to examine placebo effects. This may merit consideration by future researchers interested in this topic.

REFERENCES

Beedie, C.J., Stuart, E. M., Coleman, D. A., Foad, A. J. (2006). Placebo effects of caffeine on cycling performance. *Medicine and Science in Sports and Exercise,* 38, 2159-2164.

Borg, G. (1970). Perceived exertion as an indicator of somatic stress. *Scandinavian Journal of Rehabilitation Medicine,* 2, 92-98.

Clark, V. R., Hopkins, W. G., Hawley, J. A., Burke, L. M. (2000). Placebo effect of carbohydrate feeding during a 4KM cycling time trial. *Medicine and Science in Sports and Exercise,* 32, 1642-1647.

Docherty, M., Smith, P. M. (2005). Effect of caffeine ingestion on ratings of perceived exertion during and after exercise: A meta-analysis. *Scandinavian Journal of Science and Medicine in Sports*, 15, 69-78.

Duncan, M. J., Lyons, M., Hankey, J. (2009). Placebo effects of caffeine on short-term resistance exercise to failure. *International Journal of Sports Physiology and Performance*, 4, 244-253.

Fillmore, M., Vogel-Sprott, M. (1992). Expected effect of caffeine on motor performance predicts the type of response to placebo. *Psychopharmacology*, 106, 209-214.

Foad, A., Beedie, C. J., Coleman, D. (2008). Pharmacological and psychological effects of caffeine ingestion in 40km cycling performance. *Medicine and Science in Sports and Exercise*, 40, 158-165.

Graham, T. (2001) Caffeine and exercise: metabolism, endurance and performance. *Sports Medicine*, 31, 705-807.

Strand, B., Wilson, R. (1993) *Assessing Sport Skill*. Champaign, Ill: Human Kinetics.

In: Trends in Human Performance Research
Editors: M. Duncan and M. Lyons

ISBN: 978-1-61668-591-1
© 2010 Nova Science Publishers, Inc.

Chapter 2

THE EFFECT OF USING HIKING POLES ON O_2 UPTAKE, HEART RATE AND BLOOD LACTATE DURING UPHILL WALKING

Joseph Moreton[1] and Michael J. Duncan[2]*
Newman University College, UK
Coventry University, UK

ABSTRACT

The purpose of the present study was to compare the use of hiking poles on physiological responses to walking at various uphill gradients. This was conducted on a treadmill at various inclined gradients (0, 10 and 20%). Ten participants (mean age = 26 ± .5 years) walked for 15 minutes at 0, 10 and 20% gradients, on two separate occasions, once with hiking poles and once without in a randomised order. Participants carried a backpack weighing 9.5kg during all trials. Oxygen uptake, heart rate, blood lactate and rate of perceived exertion were assessed throughout. A 2 (conditions) X 3 (gradients) way repeated measures ANOVA was used to examine the differences in each variable across conditions. Results

---

* Please address correspondence and requests for reprints to
Joseph Moreton,
Newman University College,
Bartley Green, Birmingham, United Kingdom, B32 3NT
E mail j.moreton@newman.ac.uk

indicated that there were no significant differences in oxygen uptake ($F_{1,9} = 1.98$, $P = 1.93$), blood lactate ($F_{1,5} = 3.65$, $P = 0.572$), heart rate ($F_{1,8} = 6.827$, $P = 0.732$) or RPE ($F_{1,9} = 1.095$, $P = 0.323$) when comparing the poles condition to the no-poles condition. The results suggest that using hiking poles with respect to varying uphill gradients may not cause the increased work rate as some research suggests. However, conclusions are limited due to the ecological validity of walking on a treadmill, as opposed to an ecologically valid environment.

Keywords: Uphill walking, Load carriage, O_2 uptake.

INTRODUCTION

Hiking poles are widely used to combat the stress of prolonged walking and to aid stability. Research appears to be equivocal as to whether using poles is physiologically beneficial, particularly when walking uphill. This is important as poles may aid the ability to sustain the activity and prevent fatigue (Ainslie et al., 2005).

Some studies have reported higher O_2 uptake when walking with poles compared to without. Porcari et al. (1997) found oxygen uptake was 23% higher when walking with poles compared to without, however they conceded problems with participants self-selecting walking pace. Jacobsen *et al.* (2000) found no significant difference between the two conditions. Research has also looked at psychological measures. For example, Knight and Caldwell (2000) found that rate of perceived exertion (RPE) was significantly lower walking with hiking poles but found no significant differences in walking with or without poles in VO_2 after 60 minutes walking uphill.

Load carriage has also been employed by prior researchers as a means to simulate the sort of weight that would be carried when out walking. Knight and Caldwell (2000) used a backpack weight of 22.4kg, which seems excessive whereas Schwameder *et al* (1999) used a relatively lighter load of 7.6kg when looking at knee joint forces during downhill walking with hiking poles. Ainslie *et al* (2005) used a pack weighing 9.5kg that was said to be 'consistent with hill walking' and typical of load carriage conditions found in recreational hikers.

Despite the interest in the physiological responses to walking with and without the use of hiking poles, few studies have examined the effect of varying the gradient for uphill walking. Jacobson's *et al*'s (2000) study used 1 minute walking at 10% gradient, 2 minutes at 15%, 2 minutes at 20% and 10 minutes at 25%. For mean HR, VE and VO$_2$ they found no significant difference between the two conditions using poles and no-poles. However, the duration of data collection across conditions in this study may prohibit any conclusions that can be made based on his findings. Likewise, Ainslie et al (2002) considered gradient in terms of overall terrain and measured physiological responses. However, the gradient was not quantified in their study and instead the protocol was referred as a 'mountainous walk'. Clearly, the impact of hiking poles of the physiological response to walking is not clear and prior studies have not quantified their effect across different gradients of walking. This information is of potential interest to ergonomists, scientists and recreational hill walkers and may provide guidance as to any potential benefit to the use of hiking poles. Therefore, the aim of this study was to examine the use of hiking poles and their effect on physiological demand while walking at various uphill gradients.

METHOD

Participants

Following institutional ethics approval, 10 physically active participants (mean age = 26 ± .5 years, height = 172 ± 6cm, mass = 74.3 ± 10kg) took part in the study. Each participant gave their written informed consent and completed a Physical Activity Readiness Questionnaire (PAR-Q). If any potential risks were identified, participants were withdrawn. Participants were fully aware they could withdraw from the study at any point.

Procedure

Each participant was tested on two separate occasions, once where they were required to walk with hiking poles and once without. All testing conditions were randomised. Before walking with the hiking poles, participants completed a familiarization session regarding the use of hiking poles on a treadmill.

For both conditions, the participants walked for 15 minutes at 0%, 10% and 20% gradients (total of 45 minutes walking) whilst carrying a 9.5kg back pack. Treadmill speed was kept constant at 3 km·hr^{-1}. When walking with hiking poles, the poles were adjusted to the appropriate height by ensuring that the participants elbow was at 90° while the pole was held in a vertical position and in contact with the ground (Knight and Caldwell, 2000).

Oxygen uptake (ml·kg^{-1}·min^{-1}) was assessed continuously over the 15-minute periods using the Cortex Metalyser 3B (Cortex Metaphysic, Leipzig, Germany). Heart Rate (HR) was measured using a Polar Accurex Plus heart rate monitor (Polar Electro Oy, Kempele, Finland). Ratings of perceived exertion (RPE) were obtained using the 6-20 scale (Borg, 1970). HR and RPE were assessed every 3 minutes. Blood lactate (Bla) (mmol) was assessed using a capillary blood sample taken from the fingertip and measured at rest and then after each gradient using a portable lactate scout (Lactate Scout, Arkray Ltd, Japan).

STATISTICAL ANALYSIS

A two (conditions) by three (gradients) ways repeated measures ANOVA was conducted to examine differences in O$_2$ uptake, HR, Bla and RPE across the hiking poles and no-poles conditions. The Statistical Package for Social Sciences (SPSS Inc, Chicago) version 17 was used for all analyses.

Results

Results indicated, that during the poles condition compared to the no-poles condition, there was no significant difference in oxygen uptake ($F_{1,9} = 1.98$, $P = 1.93$), Bla ($F_{1,5} = 3.65$, $P = 0.572$), HR ($F_{1,8} = 6.827$, $P = 0.732$) or RPE ($F_{1,9} = 1.095$, $P = 0.323$). Mean values for measured variables across conditions and for each gradient are presented in Table 1.

DISCUSSION

On the basis of this study, hiking poles were not found to be physiologically beneficial in terms of work rate for the walker. However, the study suggests using hiking poles with respect to varying gradients may not cause the increased work rate as some research suggests. Results of this study regarding oxygen uptake disagree with previous research by Porcari (1997) who found that oxygen uptake was 23% higher when walking with poles compared to without. However, the results of the present study do support prior research (Jacobson et al., 2000; Knight and Caldwell, 2000) that found no significant differences in physiological responses walking with or without hiking poles.

Table 1. Mean values with and without hiking poles for each gradient

Gradient	Poles				No Poles			
	O² uptake (ml kg min⁻¹)	HR (Bpm)	Bla (mmol)	RPE	O² uptake (ml kg min⁻¹)	HR (Bpm)	Bla (mmol)	RPE
0%	11.9	90	2.4	7.4	10.9	89	2.3	7
10%	19.1	107	3.5	9.6	18.3	110	3.2	9
20%	29.5	143	5.1	12.5	29.0	143	6.5	12.3

These findings may have implications when recommending the use of hiking poles to operate in a mountainous environment. If a person gained stability from the use of poles, but they had to physically work much harder to operate them, the use of poles or not may prove to be a difficult decision. However, if as this study suggests, performers are unlikely to be working significantly harder physiologically when using hiking poles, then their use is even more desirable.

Despite this, the present study is not without its limitations. Like much of the previous research, physically active young people were used as participants whilst hill walking is undertaken as a recreational leisure activity by individuals across varying age ranges and levels of ability. It would therefore be interesting and beneficial to examine different age groups, in particular, older age groups. This is particularly important as during strenuous walking older walkers may be particularly prone to decreased physical and mental performance due to fatigue (Ainslie et al., 2005). If hiking poles offer any physiological or mechanical advantage it may be in these situations where their benefit comes to the fore.

It may also be of practical use to examine downhill walking. The current study focused solely on uphill walking across different gradients whereas hill walking is undertaken at varying gradients and in both uphill and downhill situations. Anecdotal evidence from regular hill walkers suggests that the stress placed on lower limbs when walking downhill is often greater and so testing the physiological demand and use of hiking poles when walking downhill may be very pertinent indeed. Recent research by Perrey and Fabre (2008) examined exertion level during uphill, level and downhill walking with and without hiking poles. They found VO_2 and energy cost increased with the use of hiking poles only during downhill trials. They did not report these differences during level and uphill walking. Therefore, to develop the current study, examining various downhill and uphill gradients may prove to be very informative.

It is also important to consider that the action of walking and using hiking poles on the treadmill is not the same as in the field and so there is a compromise in terms of ecological validity. In field conditions, greater differences in physiological demand may have been found. The varying terrain found on a typical hill walk may allow for more effective pole use due to the pole-to-ground interaction. Therefore, until researchers examine the impact of hiking poles on physiological and mechanical function in ecologically valid environments and during prolonged walking, the conclusions that can be drawn from this study are limited to the laboratory.

REFERENCES

Ainslie, P., Campbell, I., Lambert, J., MacLaren, D. & Reilly, T. (2005). Physiological and metabolic aspects of very prolonged exercise with particular reference to hill walking. *Sports Medicine*, 35, 619-647.

Borg, G., (1970). Perceived exertion as an indicator of somatic stress. *Scandinavian Journal of Rehabilitation Medicine.* 2: 92-98.

Jacobson, B. H., Wright, T. & Dugan, B. (2000). Load carriage energy expenditure with and without hiking poles during inclined walking. *International Journal of Sports Medicine*, 21, 356-359.

Knight, C. A. & Caldwell, G. E. (2000). Muscular and metabolic costs of uphill backpacking: Are hiking poles beneficial? *Medicine and Science in Sports and Exercise,* 32, 2093-2101.

Perrey, S. & Fabre, N. (2008). Exertion during uphill, level and downhill walking with and without hiking poles. *Journal of Sports Science and Medicine*, 7, 32-38.

Porcari, J., Hendrickson, T., Walter, P., Terry, L. & Walsko, G. (1997). The physiological response to walking with and without power poles on treadmill exercise. *Research Quarterly for Exercise and Sport*, 68, 161-166.

Schwameder, H., Roithner, R., Muller, E., Niessen, W. & Raschner, C. (1999). Knee joint forces during down hill walking with hiking poles. *Journal of Sport Sciences*, 17, 969-978.

In: Trends in Human Performance Research
Editors: M. Duncan and M. Lyons

ISBN: 978-1-61668-591-1
© 2010 Nova Science Publishers, Inc.

Chapter 3

ANTHROPOMETRIC PROFILES OF ELITE JUNIOR ICE-HOCKEY PLAYERS

Joanne Hankey[1]*, Mark Lyons[2] and Michael J. Duncan[3]
Newman University College, UK
Newman University College, UK
Coventry University, UK

ABSTRACT

The objectives of the present study were to investigate the anthropometric characteristics of elite Junior ice-hockey players. Eighteen ice-hockey players from a British 'Elite Hockey League' academy (mean age ± S.D. = 15.8 ± 1.2 years) were assessed on a number of anthropometric variables. Somatotype was assessed using the Heath-Carter method and body composition (% body fat) was assessed using surface anthropometry. Results indicated that defencemen were significantly taller than the forwards ($P = 0.009$), had greater body mass and a higher percent body fat compared to the forwards. These were not significantly different ($P > 0.05$), however the difference in body mass represented a large effect ($d = 0.83$). Defencemen were also significantly

---

* Please address correspondence and requests for reprints to Joanne Hankey, Department of Physical Education and Sports Studies,
Newman University College,
Bartley Green, Birmingham, United Kingdom, B32 3NT
Email: j.hankey@newman.ac.uk

more endomorphic (P = 0.047) than forwards, Overall, defencemen were classed as endomorphic mesomorphs and forwards were classified as ectomorphic mesomorphs. These results indicate the need for sports scientists and conditioning professionals to take the kinathropometric characteristics of ice-hockey players into account when designing individualised position specific training programmes.

Keywords: Somatotype, Anthropometry, Body Fatness.

INTRODUCTION

Ice hockey has been characterised as a high-intensity intermittent sport that includes many rapid changes in direction and velocity, as well as frequent body contacts with both the opposition and boards (Montgomery, 2000). However, there is a dearth of information relating to the physiological characteristics that are associated with high-level ice-hockey performance (Duncan, & Lyons, 2009).

Physiological assessment of athletes is important in establishing the pre requisites for successful participation in any given sport (Gualdi-Russo, & Zaccagni, 2001). In a review of ice hockey, Montgomery (2000) suggested that the physiological attributes of an ice hockey player will define their style of play and their potential for success. In addition to this, it has been commonly found that there physiological differences between playing positions in many sports (Gualdi-Russo, & Zaccagni, 2001). For example, in a study by Renger (1994), National Hockey League scouts were asked to rank the 10 task requirements on which players are assessed and assign the relative importance of each task. Shooting/scoring was weighted significantly higher for forwards, whilst checking, size/strength and positional play was weighted more heavily for defensemen. Therefore the task requirements necessary for success in elite hockey vary between positions.

Studies on positional differences in physical characteristics (e.g. through somatotype analysis) amongst male ice hockey players are limited, particularly with adolescent players (Geithner et al., 2006; Duncan, & Lyons, 2009). Recently, Duncan & Lyons (2009) examined the kinathropometric profile of British adult male ice-hockey players and reported that defencemen were more endomorphic, mesomorphic, had greater body mass and higher percent body fat compared to forwards. Duncan & Lyons (2009) suggested that these positional differences were due to differing technical and tactical demands between defence and forwards in ice-hockey. However, Duncan & Lyons (2009) highlighted a need for further research examining positional differences in anthropometric and physiological variables specific to ice-hockey. However, few data exist documenting the kinanthropometric profiles of elite junior ice-hockey players. As understanding position-specific demands within a sport is important for athlete preparation, ensuring effective training (Geithner et al., 2006) and talent identification, the aim of this study was to examine positional differences in the anthropometric profiles of adolescent, male ice-hockey players.

METHOD

Participants

Twenty male, academy ice-hockey players (mean age ± S.D. = 15.8 ± 1.24 years) participated in this study following ethical approval and informed consent. The players comprised 10 forwards and 10 defencemen from a British Elite Hockey League Academy.

Procedure

Height and mass were assessed using a Seca Stadiometer and weighing scales (Seca Instruments Ltd, Germany). Percent body fat was assessed using skinfold measures of four sites using Harpenden skinfold callipers (Harpenden Instruments Ltd, England) and employing the Durnin and Womersley (1974) skinfold equation. Somatotypes were calculated using the Heath-Carter method (Carter and Heath, 1990). All measures were completed by ISAK accredited anthropometrists whose TEMs for the sites involved were 2% or better.

Statistical Analysis

Differences within kinanthropometric variables according to playing positions (forwards and defencemen), were analysed using independent t-tests. Cohen's *d* was also employed as a measure of effect size. Statistical significance was set as $P < 0.05$ a priori and all statistical analysis was performed with SPSS version 16.0 (SPSS INC, Chicago, IL).

RESULTS

The results of all the measures taken (mean ± S.D) according to playing position are found in Table 1. Independent t-tests indicated that defencemen were significantly taller than the forwards (t_{18} = -2.932, P = 0.009), representing a huge effect (d = 1.52). Defencemen also had greater body mass and a higher percent body fat compared to the forwards (see Table 1). These were not significantly different ($P > 0.05$), however the difference in body mass represented a large effect (d = 0.83). Defencemen were significantly more endomorphic ($t_{14.111}$ = -2.174, P = 0.047) than forwards, representing a large effect (d = 1.02). Classification of somatotypes according to the Heath-Carter method revealed that defencemen were classed as endomorphic mesomorphs and forwards were classified as ectomorphic mesomorphs.

Table 1. Summary of results (Mean ± S.D.)

	Defencemen		Forwards	
	Mean	S.D.	Mean	S.D.
Height (m)	1.78	0.06	1.67	0.09
Mass (kg)	70.10	10.63	62.15	9.43
Body Fat (%)	16.34	4.52	14.52	3.12
Endomorphy	3.35	1.27	2.35	0.71
Mesomorphy	4.60	0.63	4.80	0.78
Ectomorphy	2.95	1.26	2.65	0.75

DISCUSSION

Current findings support previous research with other athletic groups (Gualdi-Russo, & Zaccagni, 2001) as well as ice-hockey players (Geithner et al., 2006; Duncan, & Lyons, 2009), that reported positional differences in somatotypes. The differences in anthropometric variables between forwards and defensemen in the current study may be due to the different technical and tactical demands across positions. Defencemen are primarily used to 'check' opposing forwards, therefore higher body mass and greater endomorphy may increase inertia for blocking (Montgomery, 2000) and provide greater body surface area for forwards to navigate around (Duncan, & Lyons, 2009). Due to the contact nature of ice hockey, greater fat mass may provide protection during collisions with boards and opponents (Montgomery, 2000). Lower endomorphy scores in forwards may also be important as speed and agility are key to this position. These findings suggest that, in junior athletes, somatotypes differ as a function of positional role within ice-hockey and that sports scientists, coaches and strength and conditioning professionals need to be aware of these requirements. The present data add support to data previously reported on adult players (Duncan, & Lyons, 2009). However, it is not clear whether ice-hockey coaches use somatotype as a means to allocate junior players to particular positions or whether the different somatotypes seen in this study and others are a result of specific adaptation to the positional requirements of ice-hockey. Further research is needed to examine this issue in addition to determining the role that anthropometric variables play in on ice performance.

REFERENCES

Carter, J. E. L. & Heath, H. (1990). *Somatotyping – Development and Applications*. Cambridge: Cambridge University Press.

Duncan, M. J. & Lyons, M. (2009). Positional differences in the kinanthropometric and physiological characteristics of elite British ice-hockey players. In *Advances in Strength and Conditioning Research* (edited by M. J. Duncan and M. Lyons). New York: Nova Science Publishers Inc.

Durnin, J. V. G. A., & Womersley, J. (1974). Body fat assessed from total body density and its estimation from skinfold thickness: Measurements on

481 men and women aged from 16 to 72 years. *British Journal of Nutrition*, 32, 77-97.

Geithner, C., Lee, A. & Bracko, M. (2006). Physical and performance differences among forwards, defensemen, and goalies in elite women's ice hockey. *Journal of Strength and Conditioning Research*, 20, 500-505.

Gualdi-Russo, E. & Zaccagni, L. (2001). Somatotype, role and performance in elite volleyball players. *Journal of Sports Medicine and Physical Fitness*, 41, 256-262.

Montgomery, D. L. (2000). Physiology of ice hockey. In *Exercise and Sports Science* (edited by W. E. Garrett and D. Kirkendall), 815-828. Philadelphia: Lippincott, Williams and Wilkins.

Renger, R. (1994). Identifying the task requirements essential to the success of a professional ice hockey player: A scouts perspective. *Journal of Teaching in Physical Education*, 13, 180-195.

Chapter 4

THE IMPACT OF CAFFEINE CONSUMPTION ON 1000-METRE ROWING PERFORMANCE

Michael J. Duncan[*]
Coventry University, UK

ABSTRACT

Studies investigating the effect of caffeine ingestion on short-term high-intensity exercise performance are equivocal and few studies have investigated the effect of caffeine on rowing performance. The aim of this study was to investigate the impact of caffeine ingestion on short-term rowing performance. Ten males and two females (mean age ± S.D. = 22.4 ± 2.6 years) volunteered to participate in this study and completed a 1000-metre (m) rowing test on three occasions in a randomised order. The first condition was a control where no solution was consumed, 5mg kg^{-1} caffeine diluted into 250ml of artificially sweetened water was consumed in the second condition and the third condition was a placebo condition where 250ml of artificially sweetened water was consumed. In both cases, solutions were consumed 60 minutes prior to exercise testing.

---

[*] Please address correspondence and requests for reprints to
Michael J. Duncan,
Department of Bimolecular and Sports Science,
James Starley Building,
Coventry University, CV1 5FB, United Kingdom
E mail michael.duncan@coventry.ac.uk

Repeated measures ANOVA indicated that 1000m rowing time was greater in the control condition compared to the caffeine condition (P = 0.01) but there was no difference between the placebo and caffeine conditions (P = 0.11). There were no differences in peak heart rate across conditions (P = 0.79). RPE values were however, significantly lower in the caffeine condition compared to the control (P = 0.002) and the placebo condition (P = 0.01). These results indicate that caffeine ingestion may have a role in dampening the perception of exertion during short-term, high-intensity rowing performance but that improved rowing time may be a result of a placebo effect as much as the ergogenic effect of caffeine itself.

Keywords: Placebo Effect, High-Intensity Exercise, Ergogenic Aid.

INTRODUCTION

There is a plethora of research that has documented the beneficial impact of caffeine consumption on endurance capacity during prolonged and exhaustive exercise, particularly in running and cycling (Graham, 2001; Bridge and Jones, 2006). However, the evidence for caffeine as an ergogenic aid for shorter-term, high intensity exercise is mixed (Doherty et al., 2004; Woolf et al., 2008).

Some studies have reported caffeine to have a beneficial impact of short term-high intensity exercise performance (Jackman et al., 1996), bench press repetitions to failure (Astorino et al., 2007) and Wingate test performance (Woolf et al., 2008), whereas others have reported no beneficial effect when compared to a placebo (Collomp et al., 2002; Bell et al., 1998; Bell et al., 2001). For example, Green et al., (2007) reported that consumption of 6mg kg^{-1} caffeine or a placebo did not significantly influence ratings of perceived exertion, peak heart rate, or the number of repetitions to failure completed during bench press exercise. This led them to conclude that the ergogenic effects of caffeine on resistance exercise performance might be limited but future research was needed to assess the impact of caffeine on high intensity exercise. Likewise, Paton et al., (2001) reported no significant differences in 20 metre sprint (10 repeats) performance and Greer et al. (1998) reported no ergogenic effect of caffeine on Wingate test performance as a result of caffeine ingestion.

Conversely, Doherty et al., (2004) has reported higher mean power and lower RPE during 3 minutes high intensity cycling with caffeine consumption compared to placebo and Stuart et al., (2005) concluded that caffeine provided substantial benefits in simulated high-intensity team sport performance.

Recently, Burke (2009) has reported that although many studies have investigated the effect of caffeine ingestion on exercise, not all of these are suited to draw conclusions regarding caffeine and sport performance. There is therefore a need for future studies to specifically examine the impact of caffeine on actual sports performance and to establish whether caffeine ingestion results in a meaningful performance change. As caffeine is likely to result in benefits in sports lasting from 1 to 60 min, there is a need for research to better document the range of protocols and doses of caffeine that produce sport-specific benefits.

One sport where caffeine ingestion might result in performance enhancement is rowing. However, there are a dearth of studies investigating the efficacy of caffeine as an ergogenic aid in rowing performance. Anderson et al. (2000) reported that there was an improvement in 2000m rowing time by 0.7% following ingestion of 6 mg kg^{-1} caffeine and 1.3% following ingestion of 9 mg kg^{-1} caffeine in a sample of 8 competitive female rowers. They concluded that caffeine produced a worthwhile enhancement of rowing performance. Examination of split time for each 500m segment of the trial revealed that the first 500m of the 9 mg kg^{-1} condition was faster than the corresponding segment in the placebo and 6 mg kg caffeine condition. In this study there was no difference in RPE values across conditions. Although the work by Anderson et al. (2000) does provide some evidence of an ergogenic effect of caffeine they suggested further research was needed to support their claims. Furthermore, the range of caffeine used (6-9 mg kg) in their study tends to be at the higher range of caffeine consumed by athletes. More recently, Skinner et al. (2009) examined the effect of lower doses of caffeine on 2000m rowing performance in a sample of well-trained rowers. Participants ingested 2mg kg^{-1}, 4mg kg^{-1}, 6mg kg^{-1} caffeine or a placebo in a randomised order 60mins prior to completing a 2000m rowing trial. Unlike Anderson et al (2000), Skinner et al. (2009) reported no significant differences in time taken to complete 2000m or total power output across trials. They did report changes in heart rate, blood lactate and plasma caffeine across trials, demonstrating a physiological effect of caffeine. They suggested that further investigation of the impact of caffeine ingestion on rowing performance was warranted. Despite this, unlike the study by Anderson et al, Skinner et al. (2009) did not report split times. As a result no inference can be made in terms of whether the ergogenic effect of caffeine is more evident in the early or later stages of a 2000m rowing trial. Subsequently, and because competitive rowing events range from 500m and upwards, it may be of interest to coaches, athletes and sports scientists to examine the impact of caffeine on shorter term rowing performance.

Several theoretical explanations for the ergogenic effect of caffeine during high-intensity exercise performance have been suggested including increased performance due to the attenuation of fatigue (Kalmar and Cafarelli, 1999) and that caffeine may act via the central nervous system to influence perception of exertion during exercise (Davis et al., 2003; Woolf et al., 2008). However, as some studies have reported no differences in RPE with caffeine consumption (Woolf et al., 2008) and others have reported RPE differences (Collomp et al., 2002) further research is needed on this topic. Furthermore, the comparison of caffeine to a placebo, as is common in studies of this nature, may mask the potential effect of caffeine on performance due to placebo effects [3] and future studies should incorporate a baseline condition where no substance is ingested in order to identify both the biological and psychological effects of caffeine on performance (Beedie and Foad, 2009).

As a result, further research is needed on the impact of caffeine on short-term, high-intensity performance such as that encountered during rowing that takes on board recommendations regarding experimental designs suggested by other authors (Beedie and Foad, 2009). Therefore, the aim of this study was to examine the impact of caffeine consumption on 1000-metre rowing performance in moderately trained athletes.

METHOD

Participants

Following institutional ethics approval and informed consent, 10 males and 2 females (mean age ± S.D. = 22.4 ± 2.6 years) volunteered to participate. All participants had experience of rowing, were free of any musculoskeletal pain or disorders and competed in team games (rugby union, football, basketball) at university level. They were currently participating in > 10 hours week programmed physical activity including strength and endurance activities. All participants were asked to refrain from vigorous exercise and maintain normal dietary patterns in the 48h prior to testing and were asked not to consume caffeine after 6:00pm the night before testing to control for the effects of caffeine already consumed (Marlat and Rohsenhow, 1980).

Design

This study employed a within-subjects, repeated measures design. Participants were informed they were participating in a study examining consistency in rowing times and that as part of the experiment, they would be asked to perform a 1000m row as fast as they could, on three separate occasions, on a Concept 2 rowing ergometer. All participants had experience in indoor rowing as part of their regular athletic training and conditioning.

Procedures

Each participant attended the human performance laboratory on three occasions. Prior to any exercise testing, body height (m) and mass (kg) were assessed using a Seca stadiometre and weighing scales (Seca Instruments, Germany). All testing took place between 9.00am and 12.00pm and at the same time for each participant to avoid circadian variation. Conditions were randomised and consisted of a control condition, where no substance was ingested, a caffeine condition where 5mg kg^{-1} caffeine was consumed diluted into 250ml of artificially sweetened water and a placebo condition where 250ml of artificially sweetened water was consumed. Solutions were consumed 60mins before each exercise trial as plasma caffeine concentration is maximal 1 hour after ingestion of caffeine (Graham, 2001).

Before the exercise tests, the participants completed a 10-min warm up consisting of both dynamic and static stretches. The exercise test consisted of a 1000m rowing exercise. Although 2000m is the predominant distance used in the 2 prior studies that have investigated this issue, rowing race distances range from 500m upwards and as the aim of this study was to examine short-term, high-intensity exercise, a distance of 1000m more accurately reflected this. The 1000m rowing test has been used in prior studies to assess younger rowers (Mikulic & Ruzic, 2008). In addition, a 1000m rowing distance requires substantially greater anaerobic contribution compared to the 75:25% aerobic:anaerobic contribution in a 2000m race (Hagerman, 2000). Participants were instructed to row as fast as they could for the whole distance. The rowing ergometer's display was blinded to participants to avoid using this as an external pacing tool. The investigator verbally informed each participant of when to start the exercise and when they had reached the 1000m distance. The time taken to complete the 1000m distance (seconds) was taken as the dependant variable of interest in the study.

During each test peak heart rate (PHR) was assessed using heart rate telemetry (Polar Electro Oy, Kempele, Finland) and on completion of each test rating of perceived exertion (RPE) was determined using the Borg 6-20 RPE scale (Borg, 1970).

Data Analysis

Any changes in time taken to complete 1000m, PHR and RPE were analysed using one-way, repeated measures, analysis of variance (ANOVA). Post Hoc analysis using Bonferroni adjustments were performed where any significant interactions and main effects were found. Partial eta squared (η^2) was also calculated as a measure of effect size. A P value of 0.05 was used to establish statistical significance and the Statistical Package for Social Sciences (SPSS, Inc, Chicago, Ill) Version 17.0 was used for all analyses.

RESULTS

Results indicated a significant main effect for the time taken to complete the 1000m distance ($F_{2, 22} = 4.01$, $P = 0.03$, Partial $\eta^2 = .267$). Bonferroni post-hoc multiple comparisons indicated that participants completed the 1000m row faster in the caffeine condition compared to the control condition (Mean Diff = 5.667, $P = 0.01$). However, there was no difference in 1000m rowing time between placebo and control conditions (Mean Diff = 2.33, $P = 0.28$) and the placebo and caffeine conditions (Mean Diff = -3.33, $P = 0.11$). Mean ± S.D. for 1000m row times across conditions is presented in Figure 1.

Peak heart rate was not significantly different across conditions ($F_{2, 22} = 0.233$, $P = 0.794$, Partial $\eta^2 = .021$). There was however, a significant difference in RPE scores ($F_{2, 22} = 7.7$, $P = 0.003$, Partial $\eta^2 = .412$) with RPE values being higher in the placebo condition compared to the caffeine condition (Mean Diff = -1.1, $P = 0.01$) and higher in the control condition and the caffeine condition (Mean Diff = 1.16, $P = 0.002$). RPE scores were not significantly different however, between the control and placebo conditions (Mean Diff = 0.08, $P = 0.809$). Mean ± S.D. for RPE across conditions is presented in Figure 2. Mean ± S.D. of all variables across conditions are presented in Table 1.

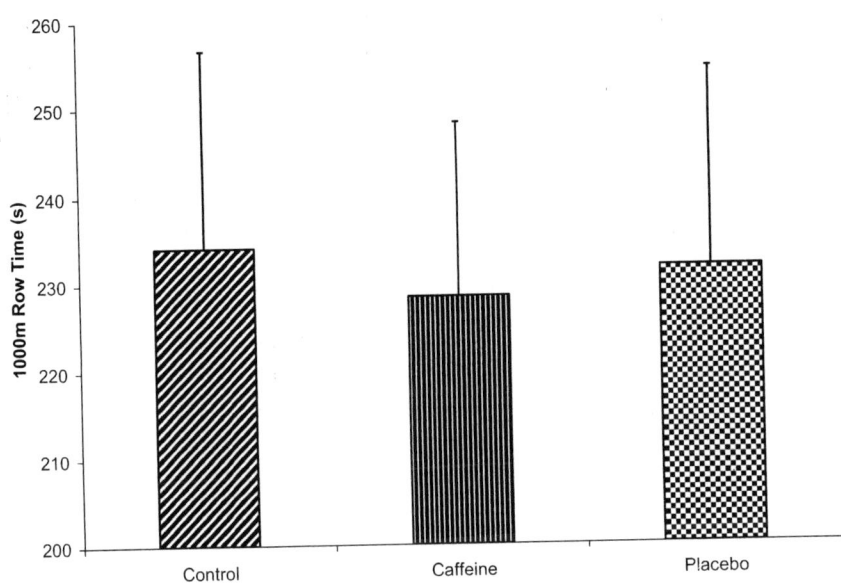

Figure 1. Mean ± S.D. for 1000m row time across conditions.

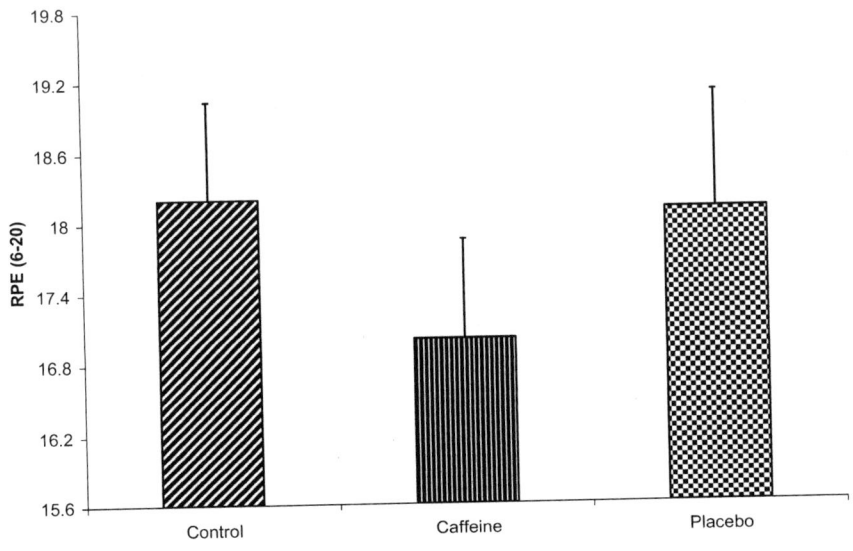

Figure 2. Mean ± S.D. for RPE across conditions.

Table 1. Mean ± S.D. of all variables across conditions

	Control		Caffeine		Placebo	
	Mean	S.D.	Mean	S.D.	Mean	S.D.
1000m Row Time (s)	234.1	22.5	228.4	19.8	231.7	22.6
PHR (BPM)	184	11.6	185	9.2	186	9.9
RPE	18.2	0.83	17.0	0.85	18.1	0.99

DISCUSSION

The results of this study suggest that consumption of 5mg kg^{-1} caffeine significantly increases performance during high-intensity rowing exercise. This concurs with previous research that has also found improved 2000m rowing time in trained oarswomen (Anderson et al., 2000) and also supports prior studies that have similarly reported increases in high intensity exercise performance, albeit not specifically using rowing performance as the dependant variable (Stuart et al., 2005; Woolf et al., 2008; Bridge and Jones, 2006). However, the results of the current study conflict with the findings of prior studies that have reported no effect of caffeine on high-intensity anaerobic performance (Bell et al., 2001; Collomp et al., 2002) and rowing performance (Skinner et al., 2009). Clearly, the results of prior studies on the impact of caffeine consumption on rowing performance are equivocal and as such inferences have to be drawn with the present study and prior studies that have used a variety of testing modalities incorporating both aerobic and anaerobic components. Due to the dearth of research specific to the efficacy of caffeine as an ergogenic aid in rowing performance further studies are warranted examining this issue specifically.

It is important to note that in the present study, the experimental design employed sought to accommodate suggestions by previous researchers (Beedie and Foad, 2009; Clark et al., 2000) regarding the design of nutritional studies and sports performance. Traditionally, this has involved comparison of an active substance (in this case caffeine) with a placebo. Beedie and Foad (2009) have noted that this design makes the assumption that the placebo is inert and does not influence performance. However, a number of studies have reported that the placebo effect can have a real and positive impact on sports performance (Beddie and Foad, 2009; Clark et al., 2000). As a result, Beedie and Foad (2009) suggested that scientists interested in examining the impact of a proposed ergogenic on performance should employ a control condition where no substance was consumed as well as the active substance and placebo conditions. In this way, scientists can determine the true physiological effect of a given substance. In the context of the current study, 1000m rowing time was significantly lower in both the caffeine and placebo conditions compared to the control condition. There was also no significant difference in rowing time between caffeine and placebo conditions. This would seem to suggest that placebo mechanisms may play some part in the ergogenic effect of caffeine on performance. It may be as Beedie and Foad (2009) note, that simply consuming a substance in the belief that it may have a performance enhancing effect, will in turn result in performance enhancement. The study of the placebo effect in sports performance is still in its infancy and further research specific to the placebo effect of caffeine on various parameters of performance is needed to verify the suggestions made based on the results of this research.

In respect of RPE values, prior authors have suggested the caffeine dampens ratings of perceived exertion during exercise (Doherty et al., 2004; Green et al., 2007) but prior research on the impact of caffeine on anaerobic performance has also reported no differences in RPE in caffeine and placebo conditions (Woolf et al., 2008). In the case of the present study, results indicated that RPE scores were lower in the caffeine condition compared to the control and placebo conditions. These findings agree with previous studies (Doherty et al., 2004; Green et al., 2007) and support the claims that caffeine ingestion reduces the perception of exertion during exercise.

Suggested Mechanisms

The potential mechanisms to explain the enhancement of exercise performance as a result of caffeine consumption have been highlighted by various authors. Ribeiro et al. (2003) speculate that caffeine might exert an effect on the central nervous system (CNS) by acting as an adenosine antagonist and blocking adenosine receptors. Adenosine inhibits the release of the most excitatory neurotransmitters in the brain and thus, caffeine blocking neuronal transmission may therefore alter perception of pain, motor recruitment and fatigue. Adenosine receptors are also abundant in skeletal muscle and the ergogenic effect of caffeine on anaerobic exercise might also stem from the antagonism of adenosine receptors (Svenningsson et al., 1997). Thus, caffeine might have a direct effect on muscle that is independent of substrate metabolism. The results of the current study would appear to support this suggestion although there is clearly a need to address this particular issue in future studies. Additional research comparing the impact of caffeine consumption on anaerobic performance across trained and untrained participants may also be useful in supporting this claim.

CONCLUSION

The results of this study suggest that consumption of a caffeinated solution increases measures of short-term rowing performance, Although this supports previous research examining the impact of caffeine on exercise performance, it also adds support to claims made regarding the placebo effect of caffeine on performance. Further research is needed to support these assertions with future authors considering a comparison of the effect of caffeine on performance in trained rowers. There is also a need for future investigation of the placebo effects of caffeine on exercise performance.

REFERENCES

Anderson, M. E., Bruce, C., Fraser, S., Stepto, N. K., Klein, R., Hopkins, W. G., & Hawley, J. A., (2000) Improved 2000-Meter rowing performance in competitive oarswomen after caffeine ingestion. *International Journal of Sports Nutrition and Exercise Metabolism.* 10; 164-175.

Astorino, T., Rohmann, R., Firth, K., & Kelly, S. (2007) Caffeine induced changes in cardiovascular function during resistance exercise. *International Journal of Sports Nutrition and Exercise Metabolism.* 17: 468-477.

Beedie, C. J., & Foad, A. J., (2009) The placebo effect in sports performance. *Sports Medicine.* 39: 313-329.

Bell, D. G., Jacobs, I., & Zamecnik, J., (1998) Effects of caffeine, ephedrine and their combination on time to exhaustion during high intensity exercise. *European Journal of Applied Physiology,* 77, 427-433.

Bell, D. G., Jacobs, I., & Ellerington, K. (2001) effect of caffeine and ephedrine ingestion on anaerobic exercise performance. *Medicine and Science in Sports and Exercise*, 33: 1399-1403.

Borg, G., (1970) Perceived exertion as an indicator of somatic stress. *Scandinavian Journal of Rehabilitation Medicine*. 2: 92-98.

Bridge, C., & Jones, M. A., (2006) The effect of caffeine ingestion on 8km run performance in a field setting. *Journal of Sports Sciences*, 24: 433-439.

Burke, L. M., (2009) Caffeine and sports performance. *Applied Physiology, Nutrition and Metabolism*. 33: 1319-1334.

Clark, V.R., Hopkins, W. G., Hawley, J. A., & L.M. Burke. (2000) Placebo effect of carbohydrate feeding during a 40-km cycling time trial. *Medicine and Science in Sports and Exercise*, 32:1642-1647.

Collomp, K., Candau, R., Millet, G., Mucci, P., Borrani, F., Prefaut, C, et al. (2002) Effects of salbutamol and caffeine ingestion on exercise metabolism and performance. *International Journal of Sports Medicine*, 23, 549-554.

Davis, J. M., Zhao, Z., Stock, H. S., Mehl, K. A., Buggy, J., & Hand, G. A., (2003) Central nervous system effects of caffeine and adenosine on fatigue. *American Journal of Physiology*, 284:R399-R404.

Doherty, M., Smith, P. M., Hughes, M. G., & Davison, R. C., (2004) Caffeine lowers perceptual response and increases power output during high-intensity cycling. *Journal of Sports Sciences*, 22:637-643.

Graham, T., (2001) Caffeine and exercise: Metabolism, endurance and performance. *Sports Medicine*, 31, 785-807.

Greer, F., McLean, C., & Graham, T., (1998) Caffeine, performance, and metabolism during repeated Wingate exercise tests. *Journal of Applied Physiology*. 85: 1502-1508.

Green, J., Wickwire, P., McLester, J., Gendle, S., Hudson, G., Pritchett, R., & Laurent, C., (2007) Effects of caffeine on repetitions to failure and ratings of perceived exertion during resistance training. *International Journal of Sports Physiology and Performance*. 2: 250-259.

Hagerman, F. C., (2000) Rowing. In: Garret, W. E., & Kirkendall, D. J. (Eds.), *Exercise and Sports Science*. Baltimore, MD: Lippincott, Williams and Wilkins.

Jackman, M., Wendling, P., Friars, D., & Graham, T. E., (1996) Metabolic, catecholamine, and endurance responses to caffeine during intense exercise. *Journal of Applied Physiology*, 81, 1658-1663.

Kalmar, J. M., & Cafarelli, E. (1999). Effects of caffeine on neuromuscular function. *Journal of Applied Physiology*. 87: 801-808.

Marlat, G. A., & Rohsenhow, D. J., (1980) Cognitive approaches in alcohol use: Expectancy and the balanced placebo design. In: NK Mello, (Ed), *Advances in substance abuse: Behavioural and Biological Research.* Greenwich, CA: JAI Press, pp159-199.

Mikulic, P., & Ruzic, L. (2008) Predicting the 1000m rowing ergometer performance in 12-13 year old rowers: The basis for selection process? *Journal of Science and Medicine in Sport,* 11: 218-226.

Paton, C. D., Hopkins, W. G., & Voillegregt, L., (2001) Little effect of caffeine ingestion on repeated sprints in team-sport athletes. *Medicine and Science in Sports and Exercise.* 33:822-825.

Ribeiro, J. A., Sebastiao, A., & deMendonca, A., (2003) Adenoside receptors in the nervous system: Pathophysiological implications. *Progress in Neurobiology,* 68: 377-392.

Skinner, T., Jenkins, D., Leveritt, M., & Coombes, J., (2009) The effects of caffeine on 2000 m rowing performance. *Journal of Science and Medicine in Sport.* 12S; S71.

Stuart, G. R., Hopkins, W. G., Cook, C., & Cairns, S. P., (2005) Multiple effects of caffeine on simulated high-intensity team-sport performance. *Medicine and Science in Sports and Exercise.* 37:1998-2005.

Svenningsson, P., Nomikos, G., Ongini, E,. & Fredholm, B., (1997) Antagonism of adenosine A2A receptors underlies the behavioural activating effect of caffeine and is associated with reduced expression of messenger RNA for NGFI-A and NGFI-B in caudate-putamen and nucleus accumbens. *Neuroscience.* 79: 753-764.

Woolf, K., Bidwell, W. K., & Carlson, A. G. (2008) The effect of caffeine as an ergogenic aid in anaerobic exercise. *International Journal of Sports Nutrition and Exercise Metabolism,* 18: 412-429.

In: Trends in Human Performance Research
Editors: M. Duncan and M. Lyons

ISBN: 978-1-61668-591-1
© 2010 Nova Science Publishers, Inc.

Chapter 5

NEW APPLICATIONS FOR ENCOURAGING FITNESS

Dorota Groffik[1] and Karel Frömel[2]*

Academy of Physical Education in Katowice, Poland, UK
Palacky University, Czech Republic, UK

ABSTRACT

The aim of the study is to verify the efficacy of pedometers in educational environments and to specify the differences between physical activity in boys and girls aged 15. One hundred four boys and one hundred fifty four girls from randomly selected classes in fourteen high schools in Katowice, Poland participated in the study. Students wore Yamax SW-700 pedometers for four weeks, continuously recorded data from the pedometers, and used motivational feedback booklets. Before and after the four-week intervention using pedometers was complemented with the IPAQ questionnaire to assess their physical activity. For statistical analysis, we used basic statistical characteristics, Mann-Whitney Test, repeated ANOVA (post hoc test Schéffe), and effect size (coefficient ω^2, d, η^2). A statistically significant difference was found between weekdays

---

* Please address correspondence and requests for reprints to:
Dorota Groffick,
Department of Theory and Methodology of Physical Education,
Academy of Physical Education in Katowice, Poland
E-mail: groffik@awf.katowice.pl

and weekend days in each week but no statistically significant differences were found between boys and girls in the average number of daily steps. After monitoring boys were more active in vigorous PA than girls, but girls more active walking than boys. No statistically significant differences were found between boys and girls in the PA declaration in IPAQ. This fact strongly suggests that the motivational properties of pedometer increase teenagers' physical activity levels. This fact is particularly evident among girls who knowing the criteria of healthy lifestyle (10,000 steps daily) are more willing to participate in the easiest form of activity i.e. walking. This is important because one can convert the number of steps into calories, and thus, can control the quantity of energy expenditure.

Keywords: physical activity, monitoring, steps, active lifestyle.

INTRODUCTION

In today's sedentary culture many in our contemporary society spends much of their time in front of televisions, computers. Regardless of how much time one spends engaged in the pursuit of audio and visual stimulation; the need for physical activity remains a primary need of one's body. A fundamental question however, remains as to what is the most appropriate and effective means of stimulating individual physical activity?

In determining which stimuli is best suited to the individual several factors should be taken into consideration. Namely, what are the physical limitations or restrictions that may limit one's choice of physical activity; what are the personal interests and goals for engaging in physical activity; and, what is the age and overall health of the individual? Clearly, one's awareness of the necessity establishing and maintaining an individually-appropriate level of physical activity is essential in developing and participating in healthy activities, and encouraging longevity.

The process of searching for possibilities to increase the level of daily, weekly and yearly physical activity should begin with children and teenagers. This is the foundation and primary goal in preparing to enjoy a healthy lifestyle. Enjoying lifelong good health concerns not only the individual activity performed during physical education classes but also the varying types of activity that may be enjoyed. Many types of physical activity are possible: normal working day activities; personal or leisure time activities: sport and recreational activities: gardening, and travel, to name a few.

According to Faulkner et al. (2008), physical activity connected with moving from one place to another is referred to as "active school transport", "active commute" (Lee et al., 2008) or "active commuting mode" (Tudor-Locke et al, 2008). The prevailing wisdom is that the foregoing defined activities have a major influence on general physical activity, especially among children and teenagers.

In this context it is "everyday-walking" which the simplest means of personal transport is; unfortunately, because of society's overall dependence on mechanized means of transport, walking is disappearing from the activities list. When diagnosing physical activity among adolescents the most important factors are sport and recreational activities in their leisure time (Kanters et al, 2008).

RESEARCH WITH PEDOMETERS

Formal programmes promoting physical activity have been shown to positively influence attitudes towards healthy lifestyles among adolescents and adults (Stone, et al, 1998). In many cases research tools are used in Physical Education classes to motivate lifelong changes in one's approach to living through an increase in physical activity (Oliver, Schofield & McEvoy, 2006; Schofield, Mummery & Schofield, 2005; Zizzi et al. 2006).

Many people use pedometers to monitor everyday physical activity. Pedometers count the number of steps taken daily, weekly, or over several months. It appears that both usability and low price have contributed to the popularization of using pedometers in schools, at work and during other individual or group activities. Historically, the interest in pedometers increased after publication of several reports on the number of steps that should be taken every day to support a healthy lifestyle. The number of steps is different for adolescents and adults. The President's Council on Physical Fitness and Sport (2005) established the Presidential Active Lifestyle Threshold of 11,000 and 13,000 steps for girls and boys, respectively. For adults, the suggested threshold is recommended as 10,000 steps, which was first promoted in Japan where the pedometers were developed and produced.

However, observations have shown that the suggested number of steps recommended in the preceding paragraph cannot be achieved by adults leading sedentary lifestyles. Unquestionably, people differ in their lifestyles and their ability to achieve pedometric goals. When establishing pedometric goals, determining the number of steps taken is essential (this is important so the interpretation of the results obtained from pedometer) can be reviewed within the context of such influencing factors as age, type of work, and physical activity. A pedometer can accurately measure the number of steps taken when walking or jogging. However, precise measurements are not possible when one is performing gym exercises.

The feature of the pedometer that has contributed most in establishing its role as a beneficial addition to one's physical fitness tools is the motivational nature of the device itself. Given that the pedometer's primary goal is to encourage the individual being tested to focus on increasing their level of physical activity, it is axiomatic that anyone can be effective in initiating changes in their lifestyle if they receive accurate, timely and personally-useful information.

Moreover, it is the self-observation that the pedometer offers which enables one to progressively increase the number of steps taken during any given day; especially on days when there is more time available to concentrate on exercise. In addition, the pedometer also contributes to the formation of physical activity routines which reinforce the need for and rewards from regular physical activity.

Recent research (Pangrazi, 2007) indicates that the most important factor in achieving one's physical fitness goals through the use of the pedometer is to set realistic and achievable goals. As an example, setting a goal of walking an additional 1,000 - 3,000 steps every day (as monitored through the use of a pedometer) establishes a baseline from which one can see progressive improvements in their level of physical activity. Through actual recording of the pedometer readings one can continue to set incremental goals in this way and create and sustain a commitment to a healthy lifestyle.

HEALTH AND PHYSICAL FITNESS

Health is a concern addressed by people of all ages. Unfortunately, some people make the conscious choice to not make health and physical fitness a personal priority, and the result can be a burden on both society (because of the tremendous cost of public health care for the infirmed) as well as the individual. Examining one's health and physical fitness needs should begin at an early age. Establishing a strong commitment to physical fitness throughout one's life will help ensure a long and prosperous life. The health literature clearly demonstrates that when adolescents make commitments to physical fitness they enjoy much healthier and longer lives.

The design and preparation of appropriate programmes based on physical activity monitoring (such as through the use of pedometers) can provide an important contribution in establishing the basis for a lifelong appreciation for, and commitment to participating in physical activity. Before any fitness program begins, it is important that one first diagnoses their present level of physical fitness.

The use of modern research equipment and techniques such as accelerometers, ActiTrainer pedometers, pulsometers and fitness questionnaire have enabled health and fitness professionals dramatically improve the information they use to counsel individuals seeking improved physical conditioning. Accordingly, it is important to explore the use of pedometers and other research techniques in the school environments, with special attention to Physical Education classes.

In the context of Physical Education classes, it is significant that when the physical activity level of both boys and girls was observed over a week long period there was a noticeable difference between the physical activity levels of boys and girls.

Recent research has focused on the characteristics and differences between boys and girls physical activity levels on weekdays and weekends. Amstrong and Welsman (2006) in their research have proven that European boys are more active than European girls. Similar results were obtained by Tudor-Locke et al (2006) who discovered that boys take more steps and are more active at weekends than girls. Additional observations on the weekly differences between European boys and girls physical activity level on weekdays and weekends were carried out by Trost et al (2000). The aspect of gender in understanding and explaining the differences between European boys and girls physical activity level of tested groups is of great importance. In most cases higher physical activity can be observed among men (Frömel et al., 2007).

Motivational capacity of the pedometer, which increases the 'walking effect', is emphasized by Zhu (2008), Welk (2008), Chan and Tudor-Locke (2008). The positive influence of the use of pedometer on the increase of physical activity among sixteen-year-old girls was observed during two-weeks of monitoring by Schofield, Mummery and Schofield (2005).

Similar results were obtained by Lubans et al. (2008) who used pedometers to evaluate after school physical activity levels among fourteen-year-old girls and boys. During the period of monitoring, an increase in the level of physical activity was also recorded.

RESULTS

The results of some noteworthy experiments carried out in primary schools prove that pedometers increase the physical activity level of tested pupils, both during the day and also during Physical Education classes (Pangazi, Beighle & Sidman, 2003). This research demonstrates the importance and necessity of introducing research tools into Physical Education classes. As has been previously indicated, pedometers assist in motivating individuals to improved physical health. It has also been demonstrated that pedometers have benefited European girls to reduce the difference between physical activity levels recorded between school days and weekends. The evidence is clear that Physical Education instructors should employ pedometers to record physical activity level of girls throughout the week.

METHOD

In our experiment 258 adolescents: 154 girls (age 15.93 ± 0.80 years, height 165.55 ± 5.83 cm, weight 55.63 ± 7.82 cm, BMI 20.30 ± 2.67) and 104 boys (age 15.49 ± 0.86 years, height 174 ±8.5 cm, weight 64.21±9.66 cm, BMI 21.13±2.59) from fourteen high schools consented and participated in the study. The classes at the schools were selected randomly. The students wore Yamax SW-700 pedometers to monitor physical activity and recorded the data in a booklet that served both as a motivational and educational resource. Each evening, the students recorded the number of steps taken, distance covered, converted it into kilometres (km) and active energy expenditure (kcal).

This research employed the International Physical Activity Questionnaire (IPAQ) (Craig et al., 2003) translated using procedures recommended by Cull et al., 2002). During the initial lesson, the students completed the IPAQ questionnaire to assess their physical activity within the last seven days. During the ensuing four weeks, the students wore the pedometers, recorded the data, and followed the instructions provided in the booklets. After monitoring their physical activity the students again completed the IPAQ questionnaire; for the second time. For statistical analysis, we used basic statistical characteristics, Mann-Whitney Test, repeated ANOVA (post hoc test Schéffe), effect size coefficient ω^2 (Tolson, 1980), d (Cohen, 1988) and partial eta squared (η^2) (Sheskin, 2007) as well as other partion analysis in Statistica 8 and SPSS 15 programs.

RESULTS

A statistically significant difference between weekday (F = 7.80; p < .001; ω^2 = .14) daily steps was found (Figure 1). The lowest average of daily steps was recorded in boys on Sunday (10390 ± 3728 steps·day^{-1}). Within the boys there was also a statistically significant differences between average steps on Friday (12829 ± 3848 steps·day^{-1}) and Sunday (10390 ± 3728 steps·day^{-1}) (p < 001, d= .63). No statistically significant differences were found in girls across the four week monitoring period. There was however, a statistically significant difference between steps on Monday (p= .025; d= .63), Friday (p= .033; d= .65) and Saturday (p= .043; d= .65) when compared to the steps of the boys. No statistically significant differences were found between boys and girls in the average number of daily steps (F=3.79; p= .053).

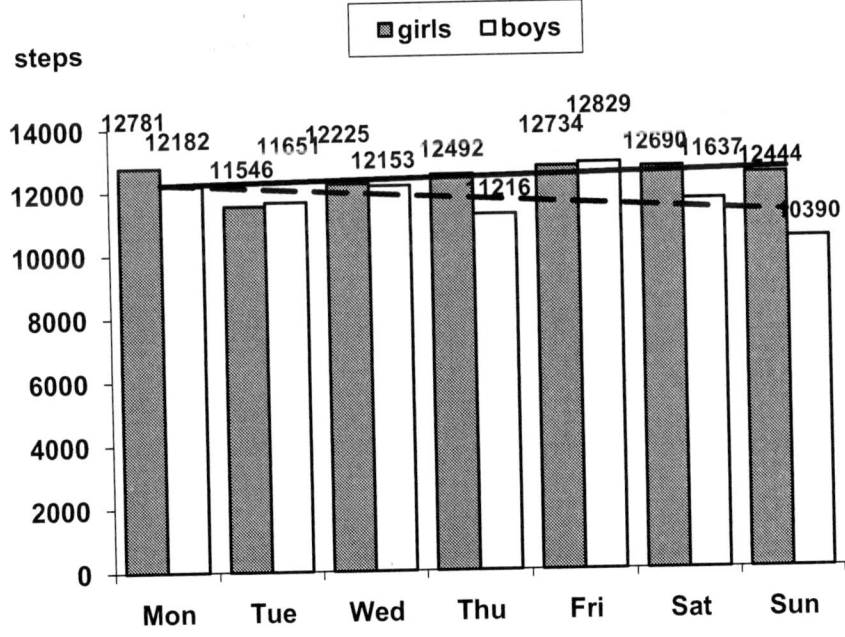

Figure 1. Average weekly step counts in boys (n=104) and girls (n=154) (steps·day-1).

A statistically significant difference was found between weekday and weekend days in each week (F = 5.46; p < 001; ω^2 = .01), but not between girls and boys. Also a statistically significant day x gender interaction was found (F=3.64; p = .001; ω^2 = .06). Girls were found to have walked more steps in the last week on weekend than boys on weekend in the first week (p = .005; d = .64) and the second week (p = .027; d = .57) (Figure 2).

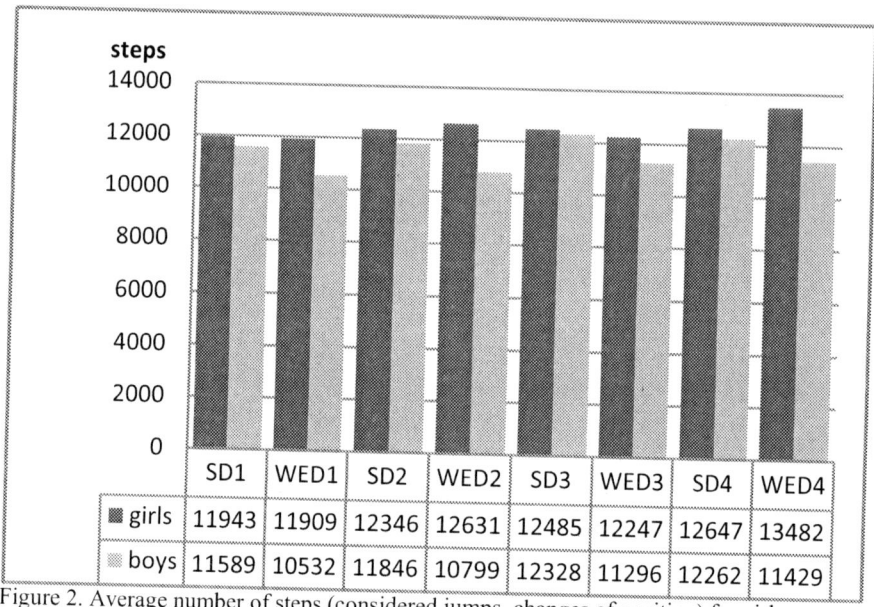

	SD1	WED1	SD2	WED2	SD3	WED3	SD4	WED4
girls	11943	11909	12346	12631	12485	12247	12647	13482
boys	11589	10532	11846	10799	12328	11296	12262	11429

Figure 2. Average number of steps (considered jumps, changes of position) for girls (n=154) and boys (n=104) in school days and weekends (steps·day-1).

Table 1. PA during weekdays (MET-min·week^{-1}) for girls and boys (pre-test)

Type/Intensity PA	Girls (n=154)		Boys (n=104)		U	P
	Mdn	IQR	Mdn	IQR		
Job	3793	4659	4494	5321	1.95	.052
Transport	1683	2310	2169	2437	.71	.478
Home	1777	2187	2456	2889	.26	.796
Recreation	2273	2370	2945	3561	1.59	.111
Vigorous	2470	3360	3261	3480	2.37*	.018
Moderate	3613	3790	5527	5812	2.48*	.013
Walk	3443	3828	3276	3564	.22	.828
Total	9525	7680	12064	10394	2.44*	.015

Note. Mdn - median; IQR – interqartile ranges; U - Mann-Whitney test
* p< .05; ** p< .01; ***p< .001

A significant difference was found between the third and fourth week and first week (F= 8,15; p < 001; ω2= .08) (Figure 3).

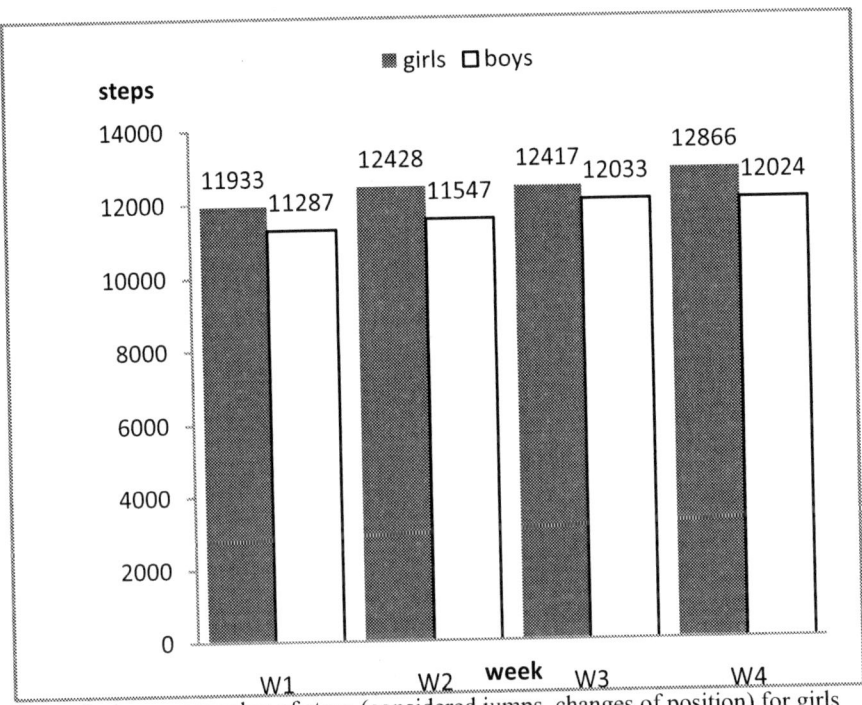

Figure 3. Average number of steps (considered jumps, changes of position) for girls (n=154) and boys (n=104) across each of the four weeks.

Prior to the start of monitoring, the boys declarations indicated that they performed more vigorous PA (U = 2.37; p = .018; η2 = .009), moderate PA (U=2.48; p= .013; η2= .010) and total PA (U = 2.44; p = .015; η2 = .009) compared to the girls (Table 1).

After the monitoring period, boys were more active in vigorous PA than girls (U=2.61; p = .009; η^2= .010), but girls more active walking than boys (U=3.13; p = .002; η^2= .012). No statistically significant differences were found between boys and girls in the all PA declarations in the IPAQ (Table 2).

Table 2. PA during weekdays (MET-min·week^{-1}) in girls and boys (post-test)

Type/Intensity PA	Girls (n=154)		Boys (n=104)		U	P
	Mdn	IQR	Mdn	IQR		
Job	2505	6084	3354	4805	1.09	.276
Transport	1944	2673	1080	2634	1.57	.117
Home	1260	2385	1087	2700	.34	.730
Recreation	2091	3024	2337	3081	.72	.471
Vigorous	**1350**	**4200**	**2580**	**2940**	**2.61****	**.009**
Moderate	3000	4500	3225	5930	1.39	.166
Walk	**3514**	**4653**	**2285**	**2821**	**3.13****	**.002**
Total	9175	10101	8781	10895	.48	.631

Note. Mdn - mediana; IQR – interqartile ranges; U - Mann-Whitney test
$p < .05$; ** $p < .01$; *** $p < .001$

The most important finding from the research conducted here is the increased level of physical activity which resulted from the experiment (steps and energy expenditure) especially within the girls.

FINDINGS AND CONCLUSION

Four-weeks of PA monitoring of high school students' did not display any vital statistical differences between boys and girls. This fact strongly suggests that the motivational properties of pedometers increase teenagers' physical activity levels. This fact is particularly evident among girls who knowing the criteria of healthy lifestyle (10,000 steps daily) are more willing to participate in the easiest form of activity i. e. walking. This is important because one can convert the number of steps into calories, and thus, can control the quantity of energy expenditure (figure 4).

The fact that girls value the usefulness and information from the experiment with pedometers more positively than boys can, in connection with other motivational factors, help increase and balance their physical activity both in school and during leisure time. The research clearly demonstrates the value of Physical Education Instructors identifying applications for the use of pedometers in girls' physical education classes.

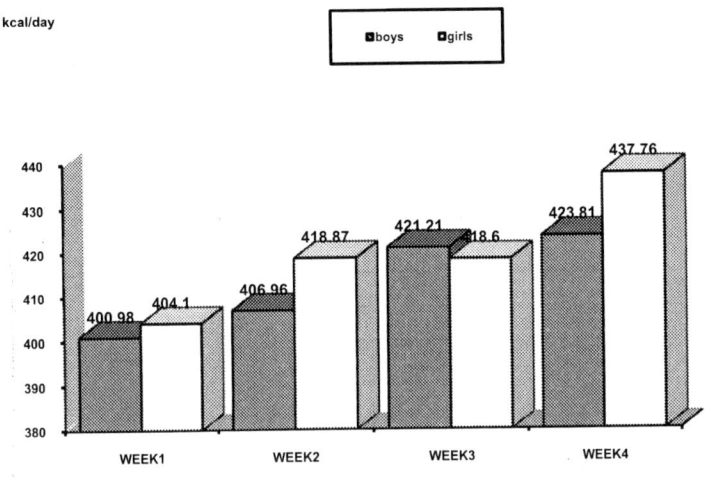

Figure 4. Energy expenditure (kcal·day^{-1}) during the four week monitoring period.

SUMMARY

In summary, it should be emphasized that pedometers provide an objective method of assessing physical activity levels, both individually and as part of group research. The results from pedometer data here, provides the basis for amending one's lifestyle and level of physical activity to enhance one's health.

Accordingly, these observed changes in physical activity can be monitored and observed in both short and long term periods. Improvements in physical activity were observed not only in over the 4 weeks but has also been demonstrated in past research (Pangrazi, et al., 2003). Official recommendations of the health benefits of properly knowing and utilizing physical fitness criteria (such as that provided by the use of the pedometer) and their positive influence on individual health can benefit the individual and society as a whole.

The National Association for Sports and Physical Education (2004) published an updated guide which establishes physical activity levels for adolescents. According to the recommendations, depending on the age of the children and teenagers referenced, these groups should be physically active for a minimum of 60 minutes to a few hours each day, preferably on all weekdays. Classes should consist of exercise of moderate and vigorous intensity (with frequent rest breaks) for the majority of the time. In addition, the recommendations encourage that everyone engage in some form of vigorous-intensity activity lasting a minimum of 15 minutes (with frequent long breaks). Extreme physical activity should be avoided, particularly during the day. The US Department of Health and Human Services (2008) also points out that adolescents should engage in aerobic exercise, at a medium or vigorous intensity, for 60 or more minutes daily. Regardless of any other recommendations, everyone should be engaged in physical activity at least three times a week.

Complimenting the US Department of Health and Human Services was a European Union recommendation on physical conditioning (EU Physical Activity Guidelines, 2008) which established similar criteria for physical activity. These recommendations were adopted in the European Union in 2006, and encouraged physical activity lasting for 60 or more minutes every day, consisting of aerobics, strength, weight bearing, flexibility, balance and motor development exercises.

However, it should be remembered that young children are spontaneously physically active and it is hard to force them to do regular exercises. It could be observed that children experience activity bursts after which there are periods of short rest. The latest research prove that this type of physical activity is appropriate for children, so it is not advisable to force them to do exercise in the same manner as adults do. Children should be spontaneously physically active for 60 minutes to a few hours.

ADDITIONAL OBSERVATIONS

It is fundamentally important in our endeavour to sustain good health to maintain a positive attitude and good physical condition. An important memory aid is the physical activity pyramid, which represents the types of physical activity in which one can engage. While similar to the food pyramid, the physical activity pyramid is somewhat different in that it consists of four levels. Each level then represents one or two types of physical activity which are directly connected to improving one's health.

The exercises which benefit people most in terms of maintaining good health are at the base of the pyramid and these are the most popular types of exercises which could be done by less active people. All kind of activities connected with everyday life such as walking, gardening, climbing the stairs are at the base of the pyramid. The recommendations accompanying the pyramid encourage participating in 30-minutes of activities which are similar to vigorously-intensive walking every day.

The first level sets forth guidelines on the easiest and the most popular type of physical activity; namely walking. Walking is monitored by the number of steps taken, distance and energy expenditure with the help of the pedometer. This is the first and most basic way to increase the physical activity. The second level of the physical activity pyramid consists of more intensive activities such as jogging, cycling or aerobics. These are exercises are more challenging, and more endurance nature. These types of exercises should be included in one's weekly workout schedule (minimum of 3 times per week, and a minimum of 20 minutes each time). The third level encompasses flexibility and strengthening exercises. At the very top of the physical activity pyramid is time at rest. This is the one level where the amount of time spent should be decreased. As stated already here, it is the tendency towards a sedentary way of living that leads to weak physical condition and ultimately a deterioration in one's health (Corbin et.al, 2007).

Knowledge of the physical activity pyramid is vital and should be applied to Physical Education classes. A different approach to physical activity is warranted due to the pace of life and the frenetic demands placed on everyone. Clearly, the goal is to persuade and convince as many people as possible that physical activity is an essential element of a healthy lifestyle. The programmes available to everyone are increasing the awareness of the importance of physical activity in everyday life. While these programs are designed for all age groups, perhaps the single-most-important is the group known as "adolescents." For healthy lives to be enjoyed young people should be convinced that physical activity is an essential part of life; and they should make it a part of their future adult life (Cavill, Biddle & Sallis, 2001). The most appropriate venue for this activity for young people is the Physical Education class where the primary goal place where such a programme should be realized is P.E. class which primary goal is to prepare and maintain a lifelong commitment to future good health through regular physical conditioning (Burgeson et al., 2001; Fairclough & Stratton, 2005; McKenzie et.al., 2006).

From a Physical Education instructor's perspective the achieving student's commitments to fitness programmes may require changes in the student's mindset and perception of the value and rewards which be achieved by engaging in exercise. Each student's physical development, attitude, and potential are different. And, in order to design and direct a worthwhile physical fitness program for each student the "individuality" of each student must be recognized. The achievement of incremental fitness goals should be reflected in such skills, knowledge and capabilities of each student in shaping the physical activity that best matches the ability of each pupil to discover the right (best) choice of exercise for their dexterity and ability.

In order to be successful the pupil and the instructor must agree on mutually realistic and attainable physical fitness goals. The student must be aware of their individual physical abilities. With the professional guidance of the instructor the student and the instructor can develop a workout routine that maximizes the interest and ability of the student with the fitness goals and schedule recommended by the instructor.

Alas, most P.E. teachers work in accordance with Motor-Fitness Performance which is focused on motor achievements (Osiński, 2000). Perhaps more important than the measure of Motor Fitness Performance which represents a more human approach to physical conditioning, is the Health-Related Fitness programme, the goal of which is to promote good health through functional efficiency and conditioning of individuals, as well as the large populations. It is recommended that Physical Education classes emphasize health improvement rather than on solely physical dexterity. The role of individual diagnosis of a physical activity and salubrious behaviour against morbidity and mortality rate is to provide knowledge essential to recognize the connection between health and lifestyle (Osiński, 2000).

Generally, the school setting promotes a healthy lifestyle for adults and adolescents (Leslie et al, 2001). Some researchers point out issues connected with the influence of problems in school setting on healthy lifestyle. In fact, some authors (Haase et al., 2004) claim that as education levels decrease, the result is a corresponding affect on salubrious education. Only 40-60% of students surveyed were aware that physical activity decreases cardiovascular diseases. Clearly, much more needs to be done. More emphasis should be placed on the promotion of healthy lifestyle against the abstract sport's results, which are sometimes achieved at a very high price.

The ability of a Physical Education instructor to diagnose the individual capacity of any student is crucial to delivering high quality instruction. From a job description perspective, the Physical Education instructor is responsible for monitoring, and directing the fitness training of the students under their supervision. With the help of the pedometer and other sophisticated measuring tools, records and questionnaires the instructor can work with all age groups to improve their overall conditioning and long-term physical fitness.

Finally, in order to enjoy a healthy lifestyle everyone who is serious about maintaining good health would benefit from learning the fundamental tips to living a healthy lifestyle, assess their level of physical activity and compare it to the standards and criteria for sustaining a healthy lifestyle. Once an individual assessment is completed one can then choose appropriate forms of physical activity that best suit their skills and ability.

In conclusion, it is of the utmost importance to consolidate and focus the knowledge about healthy living and integrate this base of knowledge with the proven methods of assessing individual physical potential. The use of pedometers, accelerometers and ActiTrainer pedometers, in evaluating physical activity levels is a very practical approach. The joining of theory and practice provides the basis for establishing a permanent commitment to regular physical activity and the lifelong conditioning benefits that result. Undoubtedly, the increase in physical activity in one's everyday life enhances not only the quality of life for the individual, but importantly the lives of everyone around them.

REFERENCES

Amstrong, N., Welsman, J. R. (2006). The physical activity patterns of European youth with reference to methods of assessment. *Sports Medicine*, 36(12), 1067-1086.

Burgeson, C. R., Wechsler, H., Brener, N. D., Young, J. C., & Spain, C. G. (2001). Physical education and activity: Results from the school health policies and programs study 2000. *Journal of School Health, 71,* 279-293.

Cavill, N., Biddle, S., & Sallis, J. F. (2001). Health enhancing physical activity for young people: Statement of the United Kingdom expert consensus conference. *Paediatric Exercise Science, 13,* 12-25.

Chan, C.B. & Tudor-Locke, C. (2008). Real-world evaluation of a community-based pedometer intervention. *Journal of Physical Activity and Health*, 5, 648-664.

Cohen, J. (1988). *Statistical power analysis for the behavioural sciences* (Second Edition). New York: Lawrence Erlbaum Associates.

Corbin, C.B., Welk, G.J., Corbin, W.R., & Welk, K.A. (2007). *Fitness i wellness. Kondycja, sprawność, zdrowie.* Wydawnictwo: Zysk i s-ka.

Craig, C. L, et al. (2003). International physical activity questionnaire: 12-country reliability and validity. *Medicine and Science in Sports and Exercise*, 35, 1381-1395.

Cull, A. Sprangers, M., Bjordal, K., Aaronson, N, West, K., & Bottomley, A. (2002). Eortc quality of life group translation procedure. Brussels: EORTC Quality of Life Unit.

EU Physical Activity Guidelines (2008). *Recommended Policy Actions in Support of Health-Enhancing Physical Activity*. Brussels, 10 October 2008.

Fairclough, S. J., Stratton, G. (2005). 'Physical education makes you fit and healthy'. Physical education's contribution to young people's physical activity levels. *Health Education Research, 20(1)*, 14-23.

Faulkner, G.E.J., Buliung, R.N., Flora, P.K. & Fusco, C. (2008). Active school transport, physical activity levels and body weight of children and youth: A systematic review. *Preventive Medicine*. 48, 3-8.

Frömel, K. et al. (2007). Physical activity in youth in the Czech Republic: Correlates of vigorous physical activity. *Ceska kinantropologie, 11(4)*, 49-55.

Haase, A., Steptoe, A., Sallis, J. F., & Wardle, J. (2004). Leisure-time physical activity in university students from 23 countries: Associations with health beliefs, risk awareness, and national economic development. *Preventive Medicine*, 39, 182-190.

Kanters, M., Bocarro, J., Casper J. & Forrester, S. (2008). Determinants of sport participation in middle school children and the impact of intramural sports. *Recreational Sports Journal*, 32, 134-151.

Lee, M.C., Orenstein, M.R. & Richardson, M.J. (2008). Systematic review of active

commuting to school and children's physical activity and weight. *Journal of Physical Activity and Health*, 5, 930-949.

Leslie, E., Sparing, P. B., & Owen, N. (2001). University campus settings and the promotion of physical activity in young adults: Lessons from research in Australia and the USA. *Health Education*, 101(3), 116-125.

Lubas, D.R., Morgan, P.J., Callister, R. & Collins, C.C. (2008). Effects of integrating pedometers, parental materials, and e-mail support within an extracurricular school sport intervention. *Journal of Adolescent Health*. 44, 176-183.

Mc Kenzie, T. L., Catellier, D. J., Conway, T., Lytle, L. A., Grieser, M., Webber, L .A., Pratt, & C. A., Elder, J. P. (2006). Girls' activity levels and lesson contexts in middle school PE: TAAG baseline. *Medicine and Science in Sports and Exercise, 38(7),* 1229-1235.

National Association for Sport and Physical Education. (2004). *Physical activity for children:A statement of guidelines.* 2nd ed. Reston, VA.

Oliver, M., Schofield, G., & McEvoy, E. (2006). An integrated curriculum approach to increasing habitual physical activity in children: A feasibility study. *The Journal of School Health,* 76 (2), 74-79.

Osiński, W. (2000). *Antropomotoryka.* Poznań: Akademia Wychowania Fizycznego.

Pangrazi, R. P., Beighle, A., Sidman, C.L. (2003). *Pedometer power:67 lessons for K-12.* Human Kinetics, Champaign, Ill.

Pangrazi, G. (2007). *Dynamic physical education for elementary school children.* Pearson Education, Inc. publishing as Benjamin Cummings, 1301 Sansome St., San Francisco, CA 94111.

President's Council on Physical Fitness and Sport (2005). *The presidents' challenge handbook.* Washington, DC: Author.

Schofield, L., Mummery, W. K., Schofield, G. (2005). Effects of a controlled pedometer-intervention trial for low-active adolescent girls. *Medicine and Science in Sports and Exercise,* 37(8), 1414-1420.

Sheskin, D. J. (2007). *Handbook of parametric and nonparametric statistical procedures.* Boca Raton: Chapman & Hall/CRC.

Stone, E. J., McKenzie, T. L., Welk, G. J., & Booth, M. L. (1998). Effects of physical activity interventions in youth. *American Journal of Preventive Medicine,* 15(4), 298-315.

Tolson, H. (1980). An adjunct to statistical significance: ω^2. *Research Quarterly for Exercise and Sport,* 51(3), 580-584.

Trost, S. G., Pate, R. R., Freedson, P. S., Sallis, J. F., & Taylor, W. C. (2000). Using objective physical activity measures with youth: How many days of monitoring are needed? *Medicine and Science in Sports and Exercise,* 32, 426-431.

Tudor-Locke, C., Hatano, Y., Pangrazi, R.P. & Kang, M. (2008). Revisiting "How many steps are enough". *Medicine and Science in Sports and Exercise,* 40(7), 537-543.

Tudor-Locke, K., Lee, S. M., Morgan, C. F., Beighle, A., & Pangrazi R. (2006). Children's Pedometer-Determined Physical Activity during the Segmented School Day. *Medicine and Science in Sports and Exercise,* 38(10), 1732-1738.

U.S. Department of Health and Human Services (2008). 2008 Physical Activity Guidelines for Americans. Be Active, Healthy, and Happy! www.health.gov/paguidelines

Welk, G.L. (2008). The role of physical activity assessments for school-based physical activity promotion. *Measurement in Physical Education and Exercise Science*, 12, 84-206.

Zhu, W. (2008). Promoting physical activity using technology. *Research Digest*, 9 (3), 1-8.

Zizzi, S., et al. (2006). Impact of a three-week pedometer intervention on high school students' daily step counts and perceptions of physical activity. *American Journal of Health Education*, 37(1), 35-40.

In: Trends in Human Performance Research
Editors: M. Duncan and M. Lyons

ISBN: 978-1-61668-591-1
© 2010 Nova Science Publishers, Inc.

Chapter 6

STRUCTURAL ANALYSIS OF BASIC LEG EXTENSOR ISOMETRIC F-T CURVE CHARACTERISTICS IN MALE ATHLETES IN DIFFERENT SPORTS MEASURED IN STANDING POSITION

Milivoj Dopsaj[1]*, Miroljub Blagojevic[2], Nenad Koropanovski[2], and Goran Vuckovic[2]

University of Belgrade, Serbia, UK
Police Academy in Belgrade, Serbia, UK

ABSTRACT

The aim of this study is to examine basic leg extensor isometric F-t curve characteristics obtained by testing in standing position. The sample consisted of 5 different sub-samples: power lifters (N=22), karate athletes (N=9), judokas (N=10), well trained athletes (N=39), and a control group

---

* Please address all correspondence and requests for reprints to:
Milivoj Dopsaj,
Faculty of Sport and Physical Education,
University of Belgrade, Department of Training Science,
St Blagoja Parovica 156, Belgrade, Serbia, Europe
E-mail: milivoj@eunet.rs

(N=31). Six contractile characteristics were investigated: F_{maxIZO} – the level of maximal isometric force; tF_{maxIZO} – the time necessary for achieving maximal isometric force; $RFD_{FmaxIZO}$ – an index of basic isometric explosive force i.e. the isometric rate of force developement; F_{relIZO} – the relative value of the achieved maximal force; $RFD_{FrelIZO}$ – the relative value of isometric rate of force developement; and RFD/F_{max} – an index which determines the level of development of basic isometric explosive force from the aspect of biological potential. Regarding all individual contractile parametres, the results showed that there is a statistically significant differences ($p < 0.001$) between the sub-samples. Regarding all standardized differences, where the criterion represented the result of control group, F_{maxIZO} in power lifters is 65.34%, in karate athletes is 11.41%, in judokas 22.58%, and at well trained population 15.12% bigger. Regarding $RFD_{FmaxIZO}$ in power lifters, the obtained value was 243.80%, in karate athletes 118.36%, in judokas 129.17% and in the well-trained group was 43.33% higher that the control group. From the point of view of RFD/F_{max} value, the obtained value in power lifters was 243.80%, in karate athletes 118.36%, in judokas 129.17% and in the well-trained group was 43.33% higher than the control group. According to the obtained analyses here related to F-t curve leg extensor characteristics, it is possible to define initial model indicators for six tested contractile characteristics in tested athletes and well-trained populations.

Keywords: Explosive force, isometric muscle force, legs extensors, isometric F-t curve characteristics.

INTRODUCTION

A key characteristic of muscles is their ability to contract or their contractile properties (Kraemer & Fleck, 2007; Milisic, 2007; Hakkinen & Komi, 1985). One of the basic contractile abilities in many dynamic and explosive sports disciplines, is the ability to generate high muscular force (in isometric – static conditions) or high muscular strength (in dynamic conditions) within short time periods (Aagaard et al., 2002; Baker et al., 1994; Haff et al., 1997; Haff et al., 2005; Hakkinen et al., 1985; Hakkinen & Komi, 1985).

Force-time curve (F-t curve) analysis has been used to evaluate skeletal muscle contractile function. F-t curve characteristics such as the rate of force developement and maximal force have been widely investigated with respect to skeletal muscle fibers, different muscle groups, different sports, ages, gender, or different training and testing methodologies (Bemben et al., 1992; Blazevich et al., 2002; Viitasala et al., 1980; Gruber & Gollhofer, 2004; Dopsaj et al., 2000; Dopsaj et al., 2001; Dopsaj et al., 2007; Mirkov et al., 2004; Pryor et al., 1994; Rajic et al., 2004; Haff et al., 1997; Haff et al., 2005; Hakkinen et al., 1985; Hakkinen & Komi, 1985). As alluded to already, a key function of skeletal muscle is the ability to generate maximal force but within a short period of time. The rate of force developement (RFD) is generally used to descrbe this ability. RFD is generally determined as the slope in the force – time curve (F-t curve) and it is calculated as a ratio of the change in force divided by the change in time – i.e. $\Delta force/\Delta time$ (Gruber & Gollhofer, 2004; Mirkov et al., 2004; Pryor et al., 1994; Haff et al., 2005; Zatsiorsky & Kraemer, 2006). A key goal of training for increasing explosiveness is the ability to generate higher RFD when performing sport-specific movements.

The leg extensor muscles are fundamental to human locomotion. The efficiency and quality of performing different movement actions during daily habitual activities or achieving in top level sport strongly depend on leg extensor muscle characteristics (Kraemer & Fleck, 2007; Nigel et al., 2008; Rajic et al., 2004; Rossignol et al., 2006; Haff et al., 1997; Haff et al., 2005; Hakkinen et al., 1985; Hakkinen & Komi, 1985; Zatsiorsky & Kraemer, 2006). One of the conditions of efficient training systems is to include valid methodological procedures which serve to evaluate general and special motor/physical abilities (Blagojevic et al., 2008; Kraemer & Fleck, 2007; Milisic, 2007; Zatsiorsky & Kramer, 2006). It is also necessary to define specific models that need physical characteristics and description. That way it is possible to establish a system of determination with known elements, which will help coaches monitor and control the quality necessary for evaluating the efficiency of training process regarding the observed period of training. The goal is to identify changes which occurred in a specific monitored training ability (Milisic, 2007; Rossignol et al., 2006; Zatsiorsky & Kraemer, 2006).

The procedure described above is even more important in multi-year preparation training systems for top athletes, where it is necessary to control the development of achieved physical abilities and the current level of fitness as a phase block of training (Issurin, 2008).

The aim of this research is to establish all basic descriptive – model characteristics of the F-t curve of legs extensor muscles as multi-joint systems responsible for locomotion in humans. That is why the standing position test was chosen as opposed to the sitting position which is common in the scientific literature (Aagaard et al., 2002; Baker et al., 1994; Viitasalo et al., 1980; Desrosiers et al., 1998; MacDougall et al., 1991; Hakkinen et al., 1985).

The aim is to measure the characteristics as integral parts – in synergy with all other muscle groups and limbs and to obtain a realistic – natural contractile potential (Blazevich et al., 2002; Kraemer & Fleck, 2007; Rajic et al., 2004).

On the other hand, sub-samples were chosen in order to define the differences between control – i.e. non-trained population, as representatives of people with natural levels of physical abilities and differently specifically trained populations. That way, according to the obtained differences of measured contractile characteristics, it will be possible to define: a) general effects of training directed in different ways; b) possible biological potentials and limits in development of the given contractile characteristics.

METHOD

Participants

The total sample consisted of 111 male subjects. The total sample consisted of 5 sub-samples representing athletes with different development levels of the monitored contractile characteristics. They are:

1) Power Lifters - PW (N=22), are athletes who overload their contractile abilities according to the maximal intensity type (force and strength aspect). Main descriptive characteristics of the sample are: (age = 23.8 ± 3.1 years, height =181.1 ± 7.3 cm, body mass = 87.1 ± 12.7 kg, BMI = 26.45 ± 2.42 kg/m^2, training experience = 5.1 ± 2.8 years). These athletes were competing at elite national level.
2) Karate athletes - K (N=9), as athletes who overload their contractile abilities according to the maximal intensity type, from the aspect of maximal speed abilities realized without any additional load. Main descriptive characteristics of the sample are: (age = 21.1 ± 2.7 years, height =179.9 ± 4.6 cm, body mass = 75.7 ± 3.1 kg, BMI = 23.41 ± 1.11 kg/m^2, training experience = 12.9 ± 1.6 years). These athletes were competing at elite international level.
3) Judokas – J (N=10) - athletes who develop and load their contractile abilities during their training sessions and match according to the maximal intensity type, and from the aspect of maximal force and strength as well as maximal speed abilities realized due to the outer resistance (the opponent's weight). Main descriptive characteristics of the sample are: (age = 22.9 ± 3.2 years, height = 184.0 ± 9.3 cm, body

mass = 88.5 ± 21.8 kg, BMI = 25.80 ± 4.00 kg/m^2, training experience = 10.3±2.9 years). These athletes were competing at elite international level.

4) Well trained population - WT (N=39) - individuals engaged in regular comprehensive physical training for at least two years, 3-4 trainings per week, 45 minutes per training session, 8 months per year. This sub-sample consisted of the second-year students in the Police Academy in Belgrade. Their main descriptive characteristics are: (age = 20.9 ± 1.1 years, height = 181.9 ± 5.1 cm, body mass = 80.5 ± 8.3 kg, BMI= 24.31 ± 2.06 kg/m^2.

5) Control group - CG (N=31) - physically active and without reported either health and other disorders or injuries. Their descriptive characteristics are: (age = 24.1±3.4 years, height = 181.5 ± 4.9 cm, body mass = 73.3 ± 7.3 kg, BMI = 22.24 ± 1.86 kg/m^2.

All tested subjects received a complete explanation of the procedures and purpose of the study and provided informed consent. The study was approved by the Ethical Committee of the Police Academy in Belgrade (Serbia).

Testing Procedure

The testing was carried out in the Special Physical Education laboratory at Police Academy in Belgrade within a two week period. All testing was conducted in afternoon hours. After a standard warm-up procedure, the subjects completed two initial trials separated by one minute (not maximal effort), for testing familiarisation purpose, and after approximately three minute of rest, they performed two trials of maximal isometric voluntary leg extensor muscle force in standing position (Dopsaj et al., 2001; Rajic et al., 2004; Figure 1[a]). There was a rest between the tested trials of at least 3 to 5 minutes (MacDougall, et al., 1991).

The testing procedure and the position of the subjects during the test is illustrated in Figure 1[a]. The subjects stood on a platform in the parallel position with their feet hip width apart and their back to the bar bearing the high sensitive tensiometric dynamometer (Program Inzinjering, Belgrade). From this position the subjects grasped the bar from behind the back at the bar-end grips, straightened their backs and went into a half-squat down to the knee angle of 130 degrees. They then attached the ring placed at the bottom of the dynamometer to the hook at the platform; the axis of the shoulder, the hand, the dynamometer and the platform hook must in the same plane perpendicular to the platform. At the sound signal the hardware-software system commenced the measurement (Figure 1[b]). The subjects performed a maximal bilateral voluntary isometric muscle force trial by trying to perform maximal intensity static attempt of extending their legs upright without changing position in either frontal or sagittal plane.

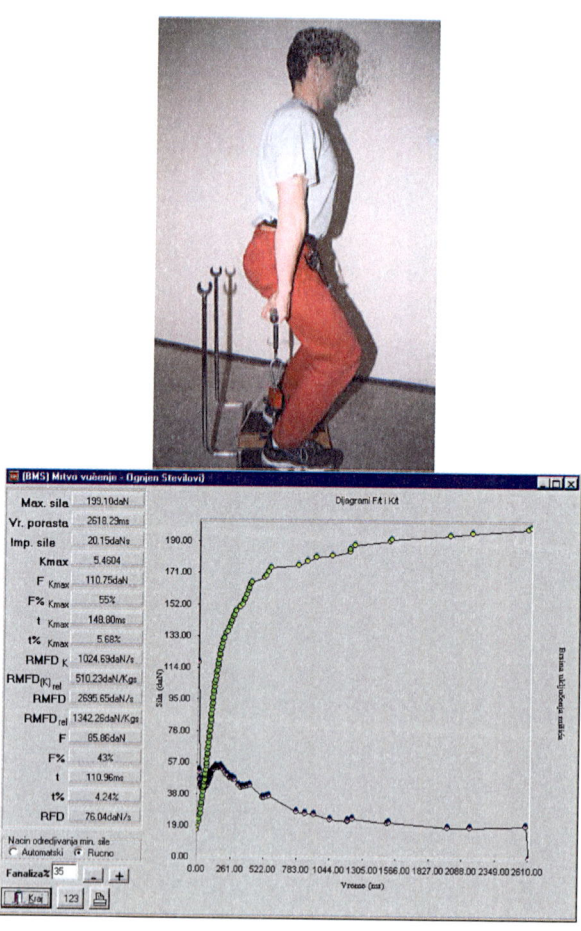

Figure 1. The position of subject during the maximal bilateral voluntary isometric leg extensor force test[a].

The testing was carried out using a high sensitive tensiometric dynamometer with maximum measurement force up to 7500 N (Program Inzinjering, Belgrade). AD conversation of force change per time units was performed at 100KHz. Thus, the obtained raw data was stored in the computer, and then the software was used to calculate the force increment per unit of time for each 1% of the force up to F_{max} level (Figure 1^b). The defined accuracy of dynamometer measurement was at the level of ± 0.1 N for force, while the accuracy of the time measurement was at the level of ± 1 ms (Dopsaj et al., 2000; Dopsaj et al., 2001; Dopsaj et al., 2007; Rajic et al., 2004).

Data Analysis Methods: F-t relations

In order to conduct this research, it was necessary to observe the following F-t curve characteristics (Bemben et al., 1992; Dopsaj et al., 2000; Jaric et al., 2005; MacDougall et al., 1991; Pryor et al., 1994; Mirkov et al., 2004; Haff et al., 2005; Zatsiorsky & Kramer, 2006):

1) F_{maxIZO} – the level of the achieved maximal isometric force, expressed in N.
2) tF_{maxIZO} – the time necessary for achieving maximal isometric force, expressed in ms,
3) $RFD_{FmaxIZO}$ – index of basic isometric explosive force i.e. the rate of force developement in isometric condition, expressed in N/s, calculated as: (F_{maxIZO} / tF_{maxIZO}) * 1000,
4) F_{relIZO} – level of achieved maximal isometric force, expressed in N/kg $BM^{0.667}$, calculated as: F_{maxIZO} / $BM^{0.667}$,
5) $RFD_{FrelIZO}$ – index of basic isometric explosive force, expressed in N^{-s}/kg $BM^{0.667}$, calculated as: $RFD_{FmaxIZO}$/ $BM^{0.667}$,
6) RFD/F_{max} – Index defining the level of the development of basic isometric explosive force from the aspect of biological potential, expressed with the index number, calculated as: $RFD_{FmaxIZO}$/ F_{maxIZO}.

Statistical Analysis

Descriptive statistics was used to calculate the following parameters: arithmetic mean (Mean), standard deviation (SD), coefficient of variation (cV%). Multivariate statistical method and General Linear Model (GLA) analyses were used to estimate general statistical differences. It was possible to define the level of difference between the tested sub-samples by using Wilk's Lambda Value. ANOVA with post-hoc multiple comparison tests (Scheffé) were performed for each observed variable separately (Hair, et al., 1998). All statistical analyses were conducted using the Statistical Package for Social Sciences (SPSS Inc., Chicago, Ill) version 11.0.

RESULTS

The GLM results have shown that there is a statistically significant difference between the sub-samples at the level of Wilk's Lambda Value - 0.171, F – 9.69, Sig. – 0.000.

Table 1. Main descriptive statistics and ANOVA results

		Power Lifters	Karatekas	Judokas	Well Trained	Control	ANOVA
F_{maxIZO}	Mean (N)	2449.34	1650.38	1815.78	1705.28	1481.36	F = 38.71
	SD (N)	378.82	157.69	468.39	225.90	241.96	P = 0.000
	cV (%)	15.47	9.55	25.80	13.25	16.33	
tF_{maxIZO}	Mean (ms)	1223.4	1304.8	1413.6	2018.3	2447.7	F = 18.49
	SD (ms)	439.3	421.4	427.2	617.8	700.6	p = 0.000
	cV (%)	35.90	32.29	30.22	30.61	28.62	
$RFD_{FmaxIZO}$	Mean (N/s)	2271.63	1442.79	1514.25	947.08	660.75	F = 34.02
	SD (N/s)	991.44	697.33	943.87	386.70	241.52	P = 0.000
	cV (%)	43.64	48.33	62.33	40.83	36.55	
F_{rellZO}	Mean (N/kg $BM^{0.667}$)	124.99	92.07	90.82	91.49	84.71	F = 25.35
	SD (N/kg $BM^{0.667}$)	16.99	8.06	12.61	10.98	13.93	P = 0.000
	cV (%)	13.59	8.78	13.88	12.00	16.45	
$RFD_{Frel\,IZO}$	Mean (N^s/kg $BM^{0.667}$)	117.56	80.78	72.42	50.80	37.97	F = 22.86
	SD (N^{-s}/kg $BM^{0.667}$)	55.27	40.42	32.42	20.43	14.72	P = 0.000
	cV (%)	47.02	50.04	44.77	40.22	38.76	
RFD/F_{max}	Mean	0.9752	0.8776	0.7948	0.5547	0.4528	F = 10.58
	SD	0.5503	0.4057	0.3319	0.2189	0.1755	p = 0.000
	cV (%)	56.43	46.22	41.76	39.46	38.77	

Main descriptive indicators with ANOVA results are shown in Table 1. The results have shown that there is a statistically significant difference between the sub-samples regarding all individual contractile parameters. The biggest difference was found in F_{maxIZO} – F = 38.71, then in $RFD_{FmaxIZO}$ – F = 34.02, p = 0.000, after that in F_{rellZO} – F = 25.35, p = 0.000, after that in RFD_{rellZO} – F = 22.86, p = 0.000, then in tF_{maxIZO} – F = 18.49, p = 0.000, while the smallest statisticaly significant difference was found in RFD/F_{max} - F = 10.58, p = 0.000 (Table 1).

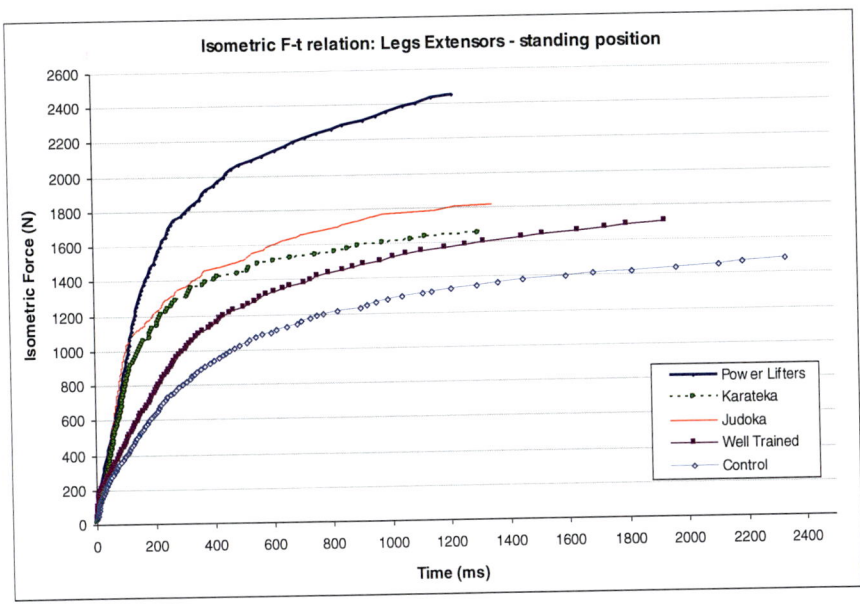

Figure 2. Isometric F-t curve for tested subsamples.

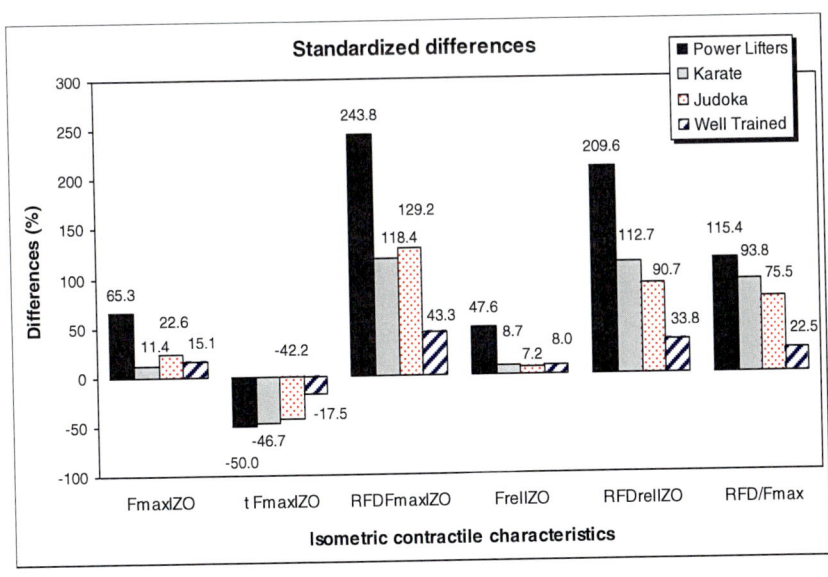

Figure 3. Standardized differences between tested subsamples according to contractile variables (dependent variable criteria - Control group).

Table 2. Multiple comparison test results (Sheffe criteria)

Sport (I)	Sport (J)	F_{maxIZO} Mean Differ. (I-J)	Sig.	tF_{maxIZO} Mean Differ. (I-J)	Sig.	$RFD_{FmaxIZO}$ Mean Differ. (I-J)	Sig.	F_{relIZO} Mean Differ. (I-J)	Sig.	$RFD_{FrelIZO}$ Mean Differ. (I-J)	Sig.	RFD/F_{max} Mean Differ. (I-J)	Sig.
PL	K	81.47		-81.45	.998	32.91	.000	84.52	.025	36.78	.086	.098	.966
	J	64.60		-190.24	.948	34.16	.000	77.23		45.14	.012	.180	.721
	WT	75.87		-794.88	.000	33.50	.000	135.07	.000	66.76	.000	.421	.000
	C	98.71		-		40.28	.000	164.26	.000	79.59	.000	.522	.000
K	J	-16.87	.818	108.79	.997	1.25	.999	-7.29	.999	8.36	.988	.083	.990
	WT	-5.60	.992	-604.64	.083	.58	.999	50.55	.319	29.98	.180	.323	.140
	C	17.24	.667	-1034.11	.000	7.37	.803	87.03	.028	42.81	.018	.425	.024
J	WT	11.27	.884	-604.64	.083	-.66	.999	57.84	.156	21.62	.465	.240	.377
	C	34.10	.045	-1034.11	.000	6.12	.340	87.03	.008	34.45	.076	.342	.092
WT	C	22.83	.041	-429.47	.061	6.78	.340	29.20	.445	12.83	.600	.102	.797

DISCUSSION

Regarding maximal isometric force the results (Table 1) revealed that the highest values during the test trial were achieved by the power lifters (2449.34 ± 378.82 N), and that it was statistically higher than all other sub-samples (p < 0.001) (see Table 2). The achieved maximal force value (F_{maxIZO}) in power lifters was 65.34% higher in karate athletes was by 11.41% higher, in judokas it was by 22.58% higher, and in well trained population it was by 15.12% higher (Figure 3). A similar structural difference has been established related to relative force values (F_{relIZO}) where the obtained value in tested power lifters was by 47.55% higher, in karate athletes by 8.78% higher, in judokas it was by 7.22% higher, while in well-trained population it was 8.00% higher than the criterion – i.e. the value achieved by the control group (Figure 3).

Regarding the time necessary for achieving F_{maxIZO} the subjects from the well-trained group had 15.77% shorter time than the control group, while judokas had by 52.25% shorter time, karate athletes by 46.69% and power lifters had by 50.02% shorter time than control group (Figure 3).

Regarding the level of general explosiveness development ($RFD_{FmaxIZO}$), power lifters were able to achieve the force generation of 2271.63 N/s with the maximal isometric leg extensor muscle contraction during the standing test. The second ones were judokas with the force generation of 1514.25 N/s, and third karatekas with 1442.79 N/s. Well-trained population followed with a force generation value of 947.08 N/s, while the control group, consisting of subjects who had not undergone any kind of physical exercise, achieved 660.75 N/s (Table 1).

It has been shown that an increase in force developement is closely related to improvements in neural drive of the trained muscles, especially in a fast dynamic, and explosive type of strength training (Hakkinen et al., 1985). The type of training used by power lifters is directed to maximal intensities and training loads related to strength, and force as the result and it is obvious that it dominantly provoked the adaptation of the organism to maximum fast and forceful muscle contraction. The adaptation influenced a higher level of $RFD_{FmaxIZO}$ which is at the level 243.80% higher than in the control population. Furthermore, the results have shown that in relation with other tested groups, power lifters have statistically significantly more developed level of explosiveness (p < 0.001) (Table 2) and it is 139.86% higher than that in the well-trained population, 57.45% higher than the karate athletes and 50.02% higher than the judokas athletes. Other authors have established almost identical results in which the highest isometric RFD values were found in male power lifting athletes who employed explosive exercises of various loads in their training (Haff et al., 1997; Hakkinen & Komi, 1985).

Regarding the indicators of relative value of general explosiveness index ($RFD_{FrelIZO}$), power lifters were able to develop 117.56 N in a second per kilogram of body mass which was divided by applying the allometric scale method ($N^{-s}/kg\ TM^{0.667}$), karate athletes could develop 80.78 $N^{-s}/kg\ TM^{0.667}$, judokas 72.42 $N^{-s}/kg\ TM^{0.667}$, well-trained population 50.80 $N^{-s}/kg\ TM^{0.667}$, while the control group developed only 37.97 $N^{-s}/kg\ TM^{0.667}$.

Although power lifters on average had the highest BMI (26.45±2.42 kg/m^2), which implies the highest body (muscle) potentials, the results have shown that they have statistically significant higher relative values ($p < 0.001$),(Table 2) of general explosiveness index ($RFD_{FrelIZO}$) by 62.34% ($p=0.036$, Table 2) regarding judokas, by 131.42 % ($p=0.000$, Table 2) regarding well-trained population. And, of course, regarding the control group, power lifters had by 209.59% higher relative values ($p < 0.001$) (Table 2) of general explosiveness level.

It is well known that some maximaly fast movement sports, as well as sprint running, karate, judo or boxing during training and competitive activities typically involve contraction times of 50 to 250 ms, or fast movement in 80 to 300 ms time intervals (Zatsiorsky & Kraemer, 2006; Aagaard et al., 2002; Baker et al., 1994; Gruber & Gollhofer, 2004).

It has been established that elite karate competitors (Koropanovski & Jovanovic, 2007) regarding the pointing way mode, most often use direct attack (38.77%), interception (23.91%) and direct counterattack (16.30%). According to pointing technique they most often win by using hand techniques (gjaku zuki cudan – 34.91, gjaku zuki dzodan – 32.00%, and kizami zuki – 16.36%). And they most often use slip (61.28%) as a type of motions in preparation to pointing or pointing attempt. They use double step (27.40%), as well. In other words, although it was established that tested karate athletes have relatively low level of F_{maxIZO} (1650.38 N, Table 1) regarding power lifters, there are no changes regarding judokas, well-trained population and control group. To be more precise, they have a lower level of F_{relIZO} than power lifters ($p=0.025$), the same level as judokas and well-trained population, and a higher level than control group ($p=0.028$). Regarding $RFD_{FmaxIZO}$, they have a lower level than power lifters ($p=0.000$), but there are no differences related to other groups (judokas, well-trained population and control group - $p=0.999$, $p=0.999$, $p=0.8.03$, respectively). However, the differences related to all but to the level of relative value of general explosiveness ($RFD_{FrelIZO}$, p=0.086) between karate athletes and power lifters has been established.

It is evident that well developed contractile ability of leg extensor muscles to develop a higher level of force per one kilogram of body mass as quickly as possible is very important for competitive success. In other words, being well-trained to move fast around the court, quick body movements, fast anticipatory movements, position adjustments and distances regarding situations during the match are the dominants for an adequate physical fitness and competitive efficiency. Since most points in karate are won by using hand techniques, in a tactful situation where we talk about hand reach, it is the explosiveness of legs in relation to the body mass of subjects that is very important as a physical ability necessary for moving fast and positioning the body in relation to the opponent.

On the other hand, the fact that during fast limb movements, therefore, the short contraction time may not allow maximal muscle force to be reached, as well as the fact that close contact in karate was not allowed during the testing, may explain the fact why karate athletes had a relatively low level of maximal leg force.

What surprises most is the fact that judokas do not have statistically significantly higher level of F_{maxIZO} (1815.78 N) in relation to karate athletes and well-trained population (1650.38 and 1705.28 N, p = 0.818 and 0.884, respectively, Table 1 and 2), as well as the level of F_{relIZO} (90.82 N/kg $BM^{0.667}$) in relation to the same groups (92.07 and 91.49 N/kg $BM^{0.667}$, p = 0.999 and 0.999, respectively) even in relation to control group (84.71 N/kg $BM^{0.667}$, p = 0.340, Table 1 and 2). Similar data were established from the aspect of explosiveness indicators as well ($RFD_{Fmax\ IZO}$ and $RFD_{Frel\ IZO}$). Obtained data may imply the fact that contractile characteristics in judo, such as maximal force level and basic explosiveness, are not too much important. However, it is believed that such way of thinking is not right and that the fact that judokas had statistically significantly higher level of the observed characteristics than karate athletes (where there were no direct contacts with opponents) than well-trained population, and even than control group, can only indicate about sensitivity and specificity of the observed variables regarding the test which was applied. In other words, it is most probable that at the level of general indicators of isometric leg muscle force, judokas need not have higher values of the characteriistics observed (the obtained level of general physical fitness satisfies all endeavors present during trainings and matches), and that they are determined and discriminated by so called specific indicators of the achieved fitness in relation to other sports (Baker et al., 1994; Blazevich et al., 2002;

Milisic et al., 2007; Nigel et al., 2008; Zatsiorsky & Kraemer, 2006). Certainly, in the future it is a must to determine the modality of the test which was applied and of the variables which were observed so that the observed characteristics of judo and karate athletes would be better determined.

After observing the index value which is defined at the level of general explosivenes development from the aspect of biological potential (RFD/F_{max}), the results have shown that in control group, as a healthy, non-trained population of the same age, it was at the level of 0.4528 (Table 1). That means that the relation between the contractile ability which defines general intensity level of isometric force development through time (explosiveness) and the contractile ability which defines general level of development of maximal minded isometric force, has achieved the ratio of 45.28%. In well-trained population, the index was 0.5547 (the ratio of these two mentioned contractile abilities was at the level of 55.47%), in judokas 0.7948 (79.48%), in karate athletes 0.8776 (87.76%) while in power lifters it was 0.9752 (97.52%).

Generally speaking, according to the data obtained in this research we can say that training labour which was applied in well-trained samples (in the period of at least two years, 3-4 trainings per week, 45 min per single training session, 8 months per year) caused higher levels of RFD/F_{max} index by 22.50% in relation to the values obtained in control group. The training labour which was applied in expirienced judokas caused an increase of the index by 75.53%, in expirienced karate athletes by 93.83% and in power lifters yet by 115.38% in relation to the values obtained in non-trained – i.e. control population.

In the previous research in which the metrological test validation was performed (Dopsaj et al., 2001) on the sample of 28 students of the second and third year of the Police Academy in Belgrade, it was established that the average F_{maxIZO} level of the subjects was 1691.45 N, average tF_{maxIZO} values were 1674.1 ms, average $RFD_{FmaxIZO}$ values were 1010.37 N/s, and that the RFD/F_{max} index was at the level of 0.5973 (59.73%). All values obtained in this research regarding the same population, categorized as well-trained individuals, are very similar to the mentioned ones, so can be considered reliable.

When general level is taken into account, and the position of all single variable values are determined in relation to the standardized multivariated Z score, the average value of the score of all variables which were observed in power lifters was at the level of 1.397, in karate athletes 0.173, in judokas 0.111, in well-trained population -0.575 and in control group -1.105. When the score is transformed into scoring system where the value of each score -3, as a hypothetical minimum expressed numerically as 0 (zero) and the value of score +3, as a hypothetical maximum numerically expressed as 100 (one hundred), then the general scoring system values are as follows: in power lifters they are at the level of 73.28, in karate athletes 52.88, in judokas 51.84, in well-trained population 40.42 and in control group it was 31.58 points.

This way, using methodologically-statistical procedure single sub-sample was located in relation to the general (multivariate) value of the observed variables which defined observed contractile abilities.

CONCLUSION

According to the obtained analyses related to F-t curve leg extensor characteristics it is possible to define initial model indicators for six tested contractile characteristics in tested athletes and well-trained population consisting of health, young and biologically mature population:

For the level of the achieved maximal minded isometric muscle force (F_{maxIZO}) of leg extensor muscles measured in standing position, where 95% confidence intervals are: Power Lifters – 2327.02 to 2571.60, Karate athletes – 1459.04 to 1841.69, Judokas – 1634.28 to 1997.32, and Well Trained 1613.39 to 1797.17 N, for lower and upper bound, respectively;

For the time necessary for achieving maximal minded isometric force (tF_{maxIZO}) of leg extensor muscles measured in standing position, where 95% confidence intervals are: Power Lifters – 975.87 to 1470.88, Karate – 917.86 to 1691.80, Judokas – 1046.51 to 1780.73, and Well Trained 1832.37 to 2204.15 ms, for lower and upper bound, respectively;

For the basic isometric explosiveness index ($RFD_{FmaxIZO}$) of leg extensor muscles measured in standing position, where 95% confidence intervals are: Power Lifters – 2012.03 to 2531.20, Karate athletes – 1036.96 to 1848.66, Judokas – 1129.24 to 1899.36, and Well Trained 754.07 to 1142.08 N/s, for lower and upper bound, respectively;

For the relative value of the level of the achieved maximal minded isometric force (F_{relIZO}) of leg extensor muscles measured in standing position, where 95% confidence intervals are: Power Lifters – 119.42 to 130.56, Karate – 83.36 to 100.78, Judokas – 82.56 to 99.08, and Well Trained 87.30 to 95.65 N/kg $BW^{0.667}$, for lower and upper bound, respectively;

For the relative value of general isometric explosiveness index ($RFD_{FrelIZO}$) of leg extensor muscles measured in standing position, where 95% confidence intervals are: Power Lifters – 104.00 to 131.12, Karate – 59.58 to 101.97, Judokas – 52.31 to 92.53, and Well Trained 40.62 to 60.98 $N^{-s}/kg\ BM^{0.667}$, for lower and upper bound, respectively;

For the value of index which defines the level of general explosiveness level from the aspect of biological potential (RFD/F_{max}) of leg extensor muscles measured in standing position, where 95% confidence intervals are: Power Lifters – 0.8365 to 1.1139, Karate – 0.6608 to 1.0945, Judokas – 0.5891 to 1.0005, and Well Trained 0.4505 to 0.6588, for lower and upper bound, respectively.

REFERENCES

Aagaard, P., Simonsen, B., Andersen, L., Magnusson, P., Dyhle-Poulsen, P. (2002). Increased rate of force developement and neural drive of human skeletal muscle following resistance training. *Journal of Applied Physiology*, 93, 1318-1326.

Baker, D., Wilson, G., Carlyon, B. (1994). Generality versus specifity: a comparison of dynamic and isometric measures of strength and speed-strength. *European Journal of Applied Physiology*, 68, 350-355.

Bemben, M., Massey, B., Boileau, R., Misner, J. (1992). Reliability of isometric force-time curve parameters for men aged 20 to 79 years. *Journal of Strength and Conditioning Research*, 6, 158-164.

Blazevich, A., Gill, N., Newton, R. (2002). Reliability and validity of two isometric squat test. *Journal of Strength and Conditioning Research*, 16, 298-304.

Blagojević, M., Dopsaj, M., Vuckovic, G. (2008). Special Physical Education I – for Police Academy students (Sec. Ed.). Belgrade: Police Academy.

Desrosiers, J., Prince, F., Rochette, A., Raiche, M. (1998). Reliability of lower extremity strength measurements using the Belt-Resisted method. *Journal of Aging and Physical Activity*, 6, 317-326.

Dopsaj, M., Milosevic, M., Blagojevic, M. (2000). An analysis of the reliability and factoral validity of selected muscle force mechanical characteristics during isometric multi-joint test. In: *Proceedings of XVIII International Symposium of Biomechanics in Sport Vol 1.* Hong Y and

Johns DP, eds. Hong Kong, Department of Sports Science & Physical Education, The Chinese University of Hong Kong, pp. 146-149.

Dopsaj, M., Milosevic, M., Vuckovic, G., Blagojević, M. (2001). Metrological value of the test to assess mechanical characteristics of maximal isometric voluntary knee extensors muscle force from standing position. *Science-Security-Police: J Police Academy-Belgrade*, 6, 119-132.

Dopsaj, M., Koropanovski, N., Vuckovic, G., Blagojevic, M., Marinkovic, B., Miljus, D. (2007). Maximal isometric hand grip force in well-trained university students in Serbia: Descriptive, functional and sexual dimorphic model. *Serbian Journal of Sports Science*, 1, 139-148.

Gruber, M., & Gollhofer, A. (2004). Impact of sensorimotor training on the rate of force development and neural activation. *European Journal of Applied Physiology*, 92, 98-105.

Haff, G., Stone, M., O'Bryant, H., Harman, E., Dinan, C., Johnson, R., Han, K-H. (1997). Force-time dependent characteristics of dynamic and isometric muscle actions. *Journal of Strength and Conditioning Research*, 11, 269-272.

Haff, G., Carlok, J., Hartman, M., Kilgore, L., Kawamori, N., Jackson, J., Morris, R., Sands, W., Stone, M. (2005). Force-time curve characteristics of dynamic and isometric muscle actions of elite women Olympic weightlifters. *Journal of Strength and Conditioning Research*, 19, 741-748.

Hair, J., Anderson, R., Tatham, R., Black, W. (1998). *Multivariate Data Analysis* (Fifth Ed.). New Jersey, USA: Prentince-Hall, Inc.

Häkkinen, K., Komi, P., Alen, M. (1985). Effect of explosive type strength training on isometric force- and relaxation- time, electromyographic and muscle fibre characteristics of leg extensor muscles. *Acta Physiologica Scandinavia*, 125, 587-600.

Häkkinen, K., & Komi, P. (1985). Effect of explosive type strength training on electromyographic and force production characteristics of leg extensor muscles during concentric and various stretch-shortening cycle exercises. *Scandinavian Journal of Sports Science*, 7, 65-76.

Issurin, V. (2008). Block periodization versus traditional training theory: a review. *Journal of Sports Medicene and Physical Fitness*, 48, 65-75.

Jaric, S., Mirkov, D., Markovic, G. (2005). Normalizing physical performance tests for body size: A proposal for standardization. *Journal of Strength and Conditioning Research*, 19, 467-474.

Koropanovski, N., & Jovanovic, S. (2007). Model characteristics of combat in elite male karate competitors. *Serbian Journal of Sports Science*, 1, 99-115.

Kraemer, W., & Fleck, S. (2007). *Optimizing strength training: Designing, nonlinear periodization workouts.* Champaign, IL:Human Kinetics.

MacDougall, D., Wenger, H., Green, H. (1991). *Physiological Testing of the High-Performance Athlete.* (Sec. Ed.). Champaign, IL:Human Kinetics.

Milisic, B. (2007). Efficiency in sport and training management theory. *Serbian Journal of Sports Science*, 1, 7-13.

Mirkov, D., Nedeljkovic, A., Milanovic, S., Jaric, S. (2004). Muscle strength testing: evaluation of tests of explosive force production. *European Journal of Applied Physiology*, 91, 147-154.

Nigel, H., Cronin, J., Hopkins, W., Hansen, K. (2008). Relationship between sprint times and the strength/power outputs of a machine squat jump. *Journal of Strength and Conditioning Research*, 22, 691-698.

Pryor, J., Wilson, G., Murphy, A. (1994). The effectiveness of eccentric, concentric and isometric rate of force development tests. *Journal of Human Movement Studies*, 27, 153-172.

Rajić, B., Dopsaj, M., Pablos Abella, C. (2004). The influence of the combined method on the development of explosive strength in female volleyball players and on the isometric muscle strength of different muscle groups. *FACTA UNIVERSITATIS: Series Physical Education and Sport*, 2, 1-12.

Rossignol, S., Dubuc, R., Gossard, J-P. (2006). Dynamic sensorimotor interactions in locomotion. *Physiology Reviews*, 86, 89-154.

Viitasalo, J., Saukkonen, S., Komi, P. (1980). Reproducibility of measurements of selected neuromuscular performance variables in man. *Electromyography and Clinical Neurophysiology*, 20, 487-501.

Zatsiorsky, V., & Kraemer, W. (2006). *Science and practice of strength training* (Sec. Ed.). Champaign, IL:Human Kinetics.

Chapter 7

ACUTE EFFECTS OF VARIABLE RESISTANCE EXERCISE ON FORCE AND POWER CHARACTERISTICS DURING THE BACK SQUAT EXERCISE

Philip H. Watkins[*] and Gareth Richards
University of Derby, UK

ABSTRACT

The use of a variable resistance (VR) combined with a traditional resistance exercise (TRE) has become increasingly popular amongst strength and conditioning practitioners as a method of training. Mostly anecdotal, the evidence has suggested that the addition of chains can improve strength and power, extend the duration of the acceleration phase and subsequently increase velocity during the concentric phase of a lift. Therefore, the purpose of this study was to investigate the combined acute effects of chain and TRE on force and power characteristics during the parallel back squat exercise. Following ethical approval and informed

---

[*] Please address correspondence and requests for reprints to:
Philip H. Watkins,
School of Science, University of Derby,
Kedleston Road, Derby, United Kingdom, DE22 1GB
E mail p.h.watkins@derby.ac.uk

consent, six recreationally trained male sport and exercise science students (Mean age ± S.D. = 22.0 ± 1.9 years) performed single, maximal effort repetitions of the parallel back squat during 3 testing sessions using the following loading conditions: Session 1, baseline measures; Session 2, condition 1- 60% of 1-RM TRE; condition 2- 60% of 1-RM TRE as well as an additional 20% of chains (VR); condition 3- 60% of 1-RM TRE and an additional 35% of chains (VR); Session 3, condition 4- 85% of 1-RM TRE; condition 5- 85% of 1-RM TRE as well as an additional 20% of chains (VR); condition 6- 85% of 1-RM TRE and an additional 35% of chains (VR). All sessions were conducted 72 hours apart to account for fatigue effects. A ballistic measurement system (Fittech, Australia) calculated force and power characteristics. One-way repeated measures ANOVA revealed significant differences ($p = 0.001$) in peak force production between TRE and all VR conditions at 60% and 85% of 1-RM. Further analysis also revealed significant increases ($p = 0.04$) in the maximal rate of force development between TRE and 60% of 1-RM and an additional 20% of chains (condition 2). The acute effects of supplementing chains with TRE may enhance acceleration during the initial concentric phase of the squat, promote power output and elevate neural drive in recreationally trained athletes. However, coaches must acknowledge the limitations in chain training until conclusive evidence is presented.

Keywords: Chains, Back squat, Resistance Exercise.

INTRODUCTION

The use of a variable resistance (VR) combined with a traditional resistance exercise (TRE) has become increasingly popular amongst strength and conditioning practitioners as a method of training. Chains and bands have become a common training technique amongst power and weightlifters and can be added to free weights to vary the external load and training stimulus (Coker et al., 2006). Chain training requires chains to be hung from the ends of a barbell which drape to the floor and used during exercises such as the squat, bench press, deadlift and Olympic lifts (Berning et al., 2008). It enables the athlete to maintain the original weight percentage for explosive training, as well as overload the top portion of the lift which normally does not receive sufficient work because of improved leverages (Simmons, 1999). Mostly anecdotal, evidence has suggested that the addition of a variable resistance can improve strength and power, enhance acceleration, elevate neural drive (Watkins and Richards, 2009) and subsequently increase velocity during the concentric phase of a lift (McMaster et al., 2009). There are limited scientific studies that support these claims (Watkins and Richards, 2009; Anderson et al., 2008; Cronin et al., 2003), whilst others (Berning et al., 2008; Coker et al., 2006) have reported no changes in kinematic and kinetic variables. Therefore, the purpose of this study was to investigate the combined effects of chain and TRE on force and power characteristics during the concentric phase of the parallel back squat exercise.

METHOD

Participants

Following University ethical approval and informed consent, six recreationally trained male sport and exercise science students (mean age ± S.D. = 22.0 ± 1.9 years; mass 78.1 ± 8.1 kg; height 176.7 ± 6.3 cm; 1-repetition maximum (1-RM) back squat 116.7 ± 14.0 kg) volunteered to participate in this study.

Procedures

A standardised warm-up preceded the performance of single, maximal effort repetitions of the parallel back squat during 3 testing sessions using the loading conditions of Wallace et al. (2006). Chain resistances (calculated from the 1-RM TRE) in this study were used *in addition* to the TRE intensity of the free weight loaded bar. All subjects underwent a familiarisation session prior to testing.

SESSION 1: Baseline Measures

Subjects were familiarised with the testing procedures, anthropometrical measures and a 1-RM assessment of the back squat exercise in accordance with the protocols of Baechle et al. (2008) was undertaken.

SESSION 2:

Condition 1 (60% of 1-RM TRE)
Condition 2 (60% of 1-RM TRE and 20% of chains);
Condition 3 (60% of 1-RM TRE and 35% of chains)

SESSION 3:

Condition 4 (85% of 1-RM TRE)
Condition 5 (85% of 1-RM TRE and 20% of chains)
Condition 6 (85% of 1-RM TRE and 35% of chains)

Chain resistances were loaded equally on either side of the barbell and attached via carabiners. Chain lengths were adapted for height differences to ensure all chain links were furled on the floor when participants reached the parallel squat position. During the concentric or upward phase, the chains were unfurled thereby increasing the resistance throughout the range of motion.

All sessions were conducted at least 72 hours apart to account for fatigue effects, and a ballistic measurement system (BMS Fittech, Australia) at a sampling rate of 500Hz calculated force and power characteristics. The BMS device was attached to the barbell for all lifts and aligned with a horizontal marker on the lifting platform. Subjects were instructed to perform lifts with their ankles above this line and the BMS cable as near to vertical at the start of each lift. The displacement setting was set to zero immediately prior to each subject performing the back squat exercise.

Anthropometry

Anthropometrical data (see Table 1) were recorded for stature and body mass using a Seca stadiometer and digital scales (Model 761, Seca Instruments, Germany). All skinfold thicknesses were obtained from the right hand side of the body, at 4 sites (i.e., bicep, tricep, subscapular and suprailiac) using Harpenden skinfold callipers in accordance with the protocols of Lohman et al. (1991).

Table 1. Participant Characteristics

Variable	Mean	Standard Deviation
Age (yrs)	22.0	± 1.9
Height (cm)	176.7	± 6.3
Body Mass (kg)	78.1	± 8.1

Statistical Analysis

A one-way repeated measures ANOVA was used to examine differences in peak force, peak power and rate of force development between TRE and all VR conditions. A Scheffè post hoc test determined the location of significant differences and effect sizes were established to ascertain their meaningfulness. $P < 0.05$ was used to determine statistical significance and the Statistical Package for Social Sciences version 16.0 (SPSS Inc, Chicago, IL) was used to perform the analyses.

RESULTS

Results revealed significant differences (p= 0.001) in peak force production between TRE and all VR conditions at 60% and 85% of 1-RM (Table 2). Further analysis revealed significant increases (p= 0.04) in maximal rate of force development between TRE and condition 2. Moderately large effect sizes (Table 3) were produced for peak force (conditions 3 and 5) and large effect sizes for peak force (condition 6) and rate of force development (condition 2).

Table 2. Statistical data for the parallel back squat across all lifting conditions

Lifting Conditions	Peak Force (N)	Peak Power (W)	MaxRFD (N/s)
Condition 1 (60% of 1-RM TRE)	1878.0 ± 255.8	2124.6 ± 383.3	3203.1 ± 1202.4
Condition 2 (60% of 1-RM TRE and 20% of chains)	1976.8 ± 279.1	2164.0 ± 588.2	4301.1 ± 1239.5
Condition 3 (60% of 1-RM TRE and 35% of chains)	2062.9 ± 255.4	2055.3 ± 435.9	3744.7 ± 864.2
Condition 4 (85% of 1-RM TRE)	2111.3 ± 253.0	2026.5 ± 617.3	3607.8 ± 793.4
Condition 5 (85% of 1-RM TRE and 20% of chains)	2313.7 ± 323.3	1996.4 ± 820.9	4201.2 ± 1428.8
Condition 6 (85% of 1-RM TRE and 35% of chains)	2387.1 ± 317.6	1902.7 ± 830.1	4168.0 ± 650.7

Table 3. Significant differences (p<0.05) and effect sizes found across the loading conditions (chains and no chains) for the parallel back squat

Lifting Conditions	Dependent Variable	P value	Effect Size
Condition 2 (60% of 1-RM TRE)	Peak Force (N)	<0.05	0.37
Condition 3 (60% of 1-RM TRE and 35% of chains)	Peak Force (N)	<0.05	0.72
Condition 5 (85% of 1-RM TRE and 20% of chains)	Peak Force (N)	<0.05	0.70
Condition 6 (85% of 1-RM TRE and 35% of chains)	Peak Force (N)	<0.05	0.96
Condition 2 (60% of 1-RM TRE and 20% of chains)	MaxRFD (N/s)	<0.05	0.90

DISCUSSION

This study supports the hypothesis that incorporating chains with TRE to alter resistance patterns may allow for an acute augmentation in strength and power measures during the performance of the concentric phase of the back squat exercise, contradicting results from previous chain studies (Berning et al., 2008; Coker et al., 2006; Ebben & Jensen., 2002). The physiological mechanisms remain unclear, however it is likely they are related to greater fibre type IIx recruitment, neuromuscular stimulation (Anderson et al., 2008) and preferential recruitment of large motor units (Nardone et al., 1989) during the eccentric phase of the squat. Similarly, acute alterations in anabolic and catabolic hormonal responses following exercise influence muscle hypertrophy and performance (Kraemer & Ratamess, 2005) and increase concomitantly with eccentric specific exercise intensity (Yarrow et al., 2008).

Several factors may have contributed to the findings of this study. Firstly, the sample size was small, suggesting that larger sample sizes may be necessary to determine the validity of chains on performance. However, studies by Coker et al (2006) and Ebben & Jensen (2002) also used small samples but concluded that chains had no effect on performance. Secondly, the ability to generate power and force through a range of motion is largely dependent upon the maximal strength available at the weakest point of the movement (Cormie et al., 2007). This study used loading conditions based on the position of least mechanical advantage (i.e., bottom of the squat) for the primary musculature involved (Berning et al., 2004), using the chains as a means to provide additional variable resistance (Simmons, 1999). In contrast, previous methodologies (Berning et al., 2008; Coker et al., 2006; Ebben & Jensen., 2002) used variable resistances to replace percentages (e.g., 80% 1RM = 75% TRE and 5% chain) of the TRE load at positions of greatest mechanical advantage. It is possible that variable resistances used in these studies were not great enough to elicit a physiological response (Berning et al., 2008). Anecdotal reports (Simmons, 1999; 1996) have recommended additional chain resistances of at least 10-15% of 1-RM TRE, depending upon the exercise and training status of the athlete.

Future studies should investigate this and TRE over an entire percentage range of 1-RM, as well as the optimal percentage range of chain load (i.e., both upper and lower body) and early-phase hormonal responses. There is also a need for intervention studies across populations (e.g., novice and elite) and standardised assessment methods if athletes and coaches are to effectively implement chain training into strength and conditioning programs.

CONCLUSION

It was concluded that the acute effects of supplementing chains with TRE may enhance acceleration during the initial concentric phase of the squat, promote power output and elevate neural drive in recreationally trained athletes. However, coaches must acknowledge the limitations in chain training until conclusive evidence is presented.

REFERENCES

Anderson, C.E., Sforzo, G.A. & Sigg, J.A. (2008). The effects of combining elastic and free weight resistance on strength and power in athletes. *Journal of Strength and Conditioning Research*, 22, 567-574.

Baechle, T., Earle, R., Wathen, D. (2008). Resistance Training. In: T. Baechle and R. Earle (eds), *Essentials of Strength Training and Conditioning*, 3rd Edition, pp381-412, Human Kinetics.

Berning, J., Coker, C. & Adams, K. (2004). Using chains for strength and conditioning. *Strength and Conditioning Journal*, 26, 80-84.

Berning, J., Coker, C. & Briggs, D. (2008). The biomechanical and perceptual influence of chain resistance on the performance of the olympic clean. *Journal of Strength and Conditioning Research*, 22, 390-395.

Coker, C.A., Berning, J.M. & Briggs, D.L. (2006). A preliminary investigation of the biomechanical and perceptual influence of chain resistance on the performance of the snatch. *Journal of Strength and Conditioning Research*, 20, 887-891.

Cormie, P., McCaulley, G. & McBride, J. (2007). Power versus strength-power jump squat training: Influence on the load-power relationship. *Medicine and Science in Sports and Exercise*, 39, 996-1003.

Cronin, J., McNair, P.J. & Marshall, R.N. (2003). The effects of bungy weight training on muscle function and functional performance. *Journal of Sports Sciences*, 21, 59-71.

Ebben, W.P. & Jensen, R.L. (2002). Electromyographic and kinetic analysis of traditional, chain and elastic band squats. *Journal of Strength and Conditioning Research*, 16, 547-550.

Kraemer, W.J. & Ratamess, N.A. (2005). Hormonal responses and adaptations to resistance exercise and training. *Sports Medicine*, 35, 339-361.

Lohman, T., Roche, A. & Martorell, R. (1991). *Anthropometric Standardisation Reference Manual.* Champaign IL, Human Kinetics.

McMaster, T., Cronin, J. & Mcguigan, M. (2009). Forms of variable resistance training. *Strength and Conditioning Journal*, 31, 50-64.

Nardone, A., Romano, C. & Schieppati, M. (1989). Selective recruitments of high-threshold human motor units during voluntary isotonic-lengthening of active muscles. *Journal of Physiology*, 409, 451-471.

Simmons, L.P. (1996). Chain reactions: accommodating leverages. *Powerlifting USA*, 19, 2-3.

Simmons, L.P. (1999). Bands and chains. *Powerlifting USA*, 22, 26-27.

Wallace, B., Winchester, J. and McGuigan, M. (2006). Effects of elastic bands on force and power characteristics during the back squat exercise. *Journal of Strength and Conditioning Research,* 20, 268-272.

Watkins, P.H. & Richards, G. (2009). Acute effects of chains on force and power characteristics during the back squat exercise (abstract). *Journal of Sports Sciences*, 27, S105.

Yarrow, J.F., Borsa, P.A., Borst, S.E., Sitren, H.S., Stevens, B.R. & White, L.J. (2008). Early-phase neuroendocrine responses and strength adaptations following eccentric enhanced resistance training. *Journal of Strength and Conditioning Research*, 22, 1205-1214.

In: Trends in Human Performance Research
Editors: M. Duncan and M. Lyons

ISBN: 978-1-61668-591-1
© 2010 Nova Science Publishers, Inc.

Chapter 8

SENSORIMOTOR EXERCISES IN SPORTS TRAINING AND REHABILITATION

*Erika Zemková**
Comenius University, Bratislava, Slovakia ,UK

ABSTRACT

This chapter deals with the role of sensorimotor exercises in sports training and rehabilitation. Both acute and adaptive changes in neuromuscular performance due to various forms of intervention are addressed. These include serial mechanical proprioceptive stimulation, task-oriented sensorimotor exercises, and those performed on unstable support surfaces. While instability agility and resistance exercises are effective for improvement of neuromuscular performance in athletes and healthly subjects, visual feedback exercise seems to be a promising tool for retraining balance function in individuals after injury. It may be of potential use also in elderly populations, for decreasing risk of falling and reduction of health-related consequences.

Keywords: Balance Exercises, Serial Mechanical Proprioceptive Stimulation, Visual Feedback Exercises

---

[*] Please address correspondence and requests for reprints toAssoc. Prof. Erika Zemková, Ph.D.,Faculty of Physical Education and Sport, Comenius UniversityNábr. arm. gen. L. Svobodu 9, 814 69 Bratislava, Slovakia E-mail: zemkova@yahoo.com

INTRODUCTION

Balance is the ability to maintain a given posture with minimal movement sway in **static** or **dynamic conditions**. Also **stance symmetry** in terms of weight distribution between the feet in a standing position plays a role in maintenance of balance. However, it has to be taken into account that balance, in most situations, is associated with other tasks (e.g., picking up an object or kicking a ball). From this point of view, it is important to focus exercise programs on improvement of postural control in order to be flexible and adaptable to perturbations.

According to Nashner (1976) appropriate anticipatory responses to postural disturbances can be learned. Backward movement of a sliding platform tilts the body forward, calling for countervailing action in the stretched gastrocnemius to maintain balance. In successive trials the muscular response is enhanced and its latency reduced. When the platform is tilted backward, action by gastrocnemius would worsen the backward body tilt. Accordingly, in successive trials the muscle's response is decreased, with a corresponding decrease of backward sway.

Besides traditional coordination or tai-chi exercises, recently whole body vibrations became a part of athletic training and rehabilitation (e.g., Wierzbicka et al., 1998; Torvinen et al., 2002; Priplata et al., 2003; Torvinen et al., 2003; Verschueren et al., 2004). For this purpose, special exercise devices have been widely employed in sport and clinical setting. However, in the playing field or gym mainly **instability resistance exercises** (Anderson, Behm, 2005) or **balance exercises performed concurrently with a secondary reaction task** are preferred. Specific forms of exercise include squats performed on an unstable surface in an altered-G environment that have been found (Oddsson et al., 2006/a; Oddsson et al., 2006/b; Zemková et al., 2006/a; Oddsson et al., 2007; Zemková et al., 2007/b) to improve both strength and balance following 4 weeks of training in untrained subjects. These exercises may be applied mainly in pre- and in-flight regimens for astronauts and in rehabilitation of bed-ridden patients. However, our experience showed no crossover effect of such functionally directed balance training on parameters of static balance. Scarce evidence also exists whether balance exercises enhance stance symmetry.

A suitable alternative seems to be **platform feedback exercises**. For this purpose systems are being designed that provide visual or auditory biofeedback to subjects regarding the locus of their center of pressure (COP). These systems usually consist of two force plates allowing to determine the weight distribution on each foot, a computer screen allowing visualization of the COP, and software providing training protocols and data analysis. Some units allow auditory feedback in addition to the visual feedback in response to errors in performance. However, platform feedback exercises have been found (Barclay-Goddard et al., 2004) to improve stance symmetry but not postural stability in standing and clinical balance outcomes (Berg Balance Scale and Timed Up and Go).

Therefore, more sophisticated methods, namely those enabling both training and assessment of sensorimotor function are needed. More promising seems to be those closer to functional activities like **task-oriented sensorimotor exercises** performed on either a stable or unstable platform equipped with PC system for feedback monitoring of COM movement (Hamar, 2008). The advantage of the system is that can be used for training but also for diagnostic purposes. In addition, there are variety of task settings like "Hit the target" or "Trace the curve" by horizontal shifting of COM.

In the first case, subjects have to hit the target randomly appearing in one of the corners of the screen by horizontal shifting of COM in appropriate direction. The test consists of 2 sets of 20 responses while better result is taken for the evaluation. Time, distance, and velocity of COP trajectory between stimulus appearance and its hit by visually-guided COM movement on the screen are registered by means of the system FiTRO Sway Check based on dynamometric platform (www.fitronic.sk).

In the second, subjects are provided by feedback on COM displacement on a computer screen while standing on dynamometric platform. Their task is to trace, by shifting COM, a curve flowing either in horizontal or vertical direction. The test consists of three 30-seconds trials randomly performing in antero-posterior and medio-lateral direction. The deviation of instant COP position from the curve is recorded at 100 Hz by means of the system FiTRO Sway Check (www.fitronic.sk).

Analysis of repeated measures showed measurement error of 8.8% for visually-guided COM target-matching task and 7.0% for visually-guided COM tracking task, which is within the range comparable to common motor tests. Test-retest correlation coefficient between repeated measurements in different days was 0.81 for visually-guided COM target-matching task and 0.83 for visually-guided COM tracking task, which signify good reliability. Also the testing protocols were standardized by analysing of sensorimotor parameters under various conditions, e.g. using different velocity and positioning of the curve tracking by a visually-guided COM (Zemková, Hamar, 2010a).

Experience showed that these task-oriented tests, based on visual feedback control of body position, can be applied for an evaluation of sensorimotor performance in individuals of different age and expertise, as well as its changes after training and rehabilitation programs (Table 1). However, different effects on sensorimotor parameters can be observed depending on the population tested (Zemková, Hamar, 2009) and the experimental conditions used (Zemková et al., 2010).

Preliminary results showed no significant differences in parameters of balance registered during quiet standing on a dynamometric platform between dancers, students and older women. On the other hand, mean COP distance from both horizontally and vertically flowing curves was significantly lower in dancers than in students and older women. These findings indicate that for some athletes, untrained subjects and elderly people, the task-oriented tests based on visual feedback control of body position might represent a more sensitive and therefore more appropriate method allowing discrimination of **individuals of different age and performance level** than evaluation of postural stability under static conditions. Lower sensitivity of static posturography is a consequence of multiple sensory inputs (visual, proprioceptive, and vestibular) involved in postural control. This can compensate smaller impairment of the system in such a way that under normal conditions (quiet stance) no deficits in postural stability may be apparent. Under dynamic conditions (stance on unstable surface) or while performing task-oriented sensorimotor exercise, the control mechanisms is taxed to a substantially higher extent so that individual differences can be revealed.

Since there are contradictory findings on relationship between proprioceptive acuity and motor skill level, we were also interested whether highly-skilled athletes of snowboarding and windsurfing would have more precise perception of COM position and its regulation during visually-guided COM tracking task than cyclists and rowers. Therefore, we compared the accuracy of visual feedback control of COP movement in antero-posterior (A-P) and medio-lateral (M-L) direction during visually-guided COM tracking task in **athletes of different specializations**. It has been found that COP distance from both horizontally and vertically flowing curves was only slightly lower in competitors of snowboarding, windsurfing, and karate as compared to cyclists and rowers. For these athletes the regulation of COM movement based on visual feedback of its position on a computer screen likely does not represent a typical form of body control. Therefore, in order to obtain sensorimotor parameters relevant to most free-style sports, the specific test close to the one used during training or competition should be preferred. For these highly-skilled athletes, dynamic posturography seems to be more sensitive method reflecting their sport-specific adaptation (Zemková et al., 2005).

However, visually-guided COM tracking task might be an appropriate alternative for **individuals after lower limb injury,** namely in an early phase of rehabilitation when effusion and pain in a joint can make it exquisitely sensitive to movement when the joint is moved in a way that is perceived as possibly aggravating that injury. Indeed, our results showed that mean COP distance from the curve was significantly higher in antero-posterior than in medio-lateral direction while performing the test on injured leg, whereas its values did not differ significantly between both directions during standing on non-injured leg. In addition, these differences were more pronounced on ankle than knee injured leg. As regulation of body position in A-P direction is provided predominantly by ankle strategy, an increase in threshold of perception of ankle movement due to injury may be assumed. From physiology it is known that this effect may be ascribed to mainly a decreased sensitivity of receptors around the joint. It may be assumed that resulting partial reduction of afferent impulses leading to deterioration in proprioceptive feedback control of balance after injury very probably contributed to less precise perception of COM position and regulation its movement in antero-posterior direction.

Table 1. Possible testing conditions for an evaluation of sensorimotor performance in various populations

Subjects	Standing on stable surface	Performing task-oriented exercise	Standing on unstable surface
Individuals of different age and performance level	very old people and those with impaired coordination	elderly people	elite athletes
Athletes of different sport specializations Individuals after lower limb injury	e.g., shooting post-injury phase	e.g., dancing early phase of rehabilitation	e.g., snowboarding late phase of exercise program

It is also known that when the reliability of proprioceptive information is reduced, either by standing on a sway-referenced surface (Redfern et al., 2001)

or on a compliant foam surface (Teasdale et al., 1993), there is an increased attentional demand associated with maintenance of balance. Vision is of particular greater relevance when the demands on postural tasks are increased (Buchanan, Horak, 1999; Mergner et al., 2005). According to Taube et al (2008) there is a significant interaction between the visual and the support surface conditions indicating that the H-reflex is more strongly affected by changes in visual feedback during standing on unstable surface. However, there is lack of information on the role of **vision and stance support conditions** in task-oriented sensorimotor exercise.

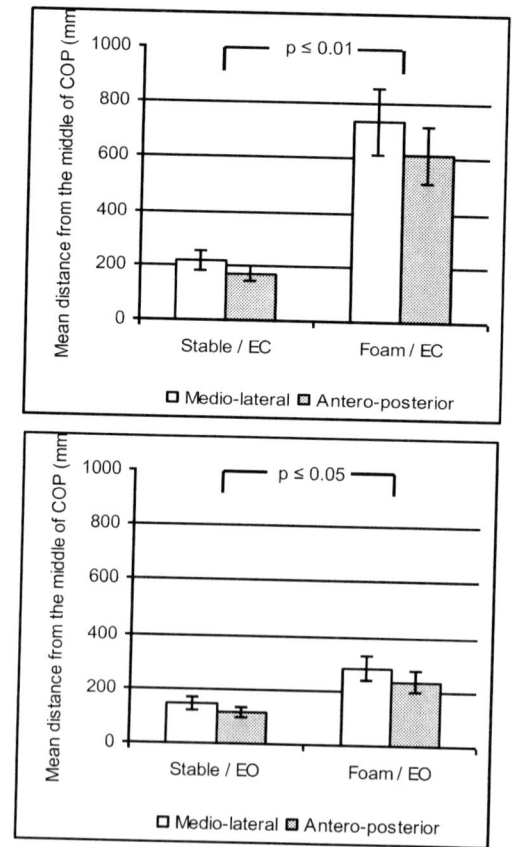

Figure 1 Mean distance from the middle of COP in M-L and A-P direction during standing on either stable or foam surface with (a) eyes closed and (b) eyes open, respectively.

Therefore, we compared the postural sway in antero-posterior and medio-lateral direction while standing either on stable or foam surface a) without visual control (EC), b) with eyes open (EO), and c) during visually-guided COM tracking task. It has been found that a deprivation of visual control and reduced stance support led to significantly ($p \leq 0.01$) higher mean distance from the middle of COP as compared to standing on stable surface with EC (Figure 1a). Its values were also significantly ($p \leq 0.05$) higher during standing on foam with EO than on stable surface with EO (Figure 1b). On the other hand, there were no significant differences in mean COP distance from the curve while performing visually-guided COM tracking task on stable and on foam surface (Figure 2). In addition, postural control was more compromised in antero-posterior than in medio-lateral direction during task-oriented sensorimotor exercise whereas opposite was true for quiet standing. It may be assumed that **visual feedback control of body position compensates for reduced proprioceptive information during standing on foam surface.**

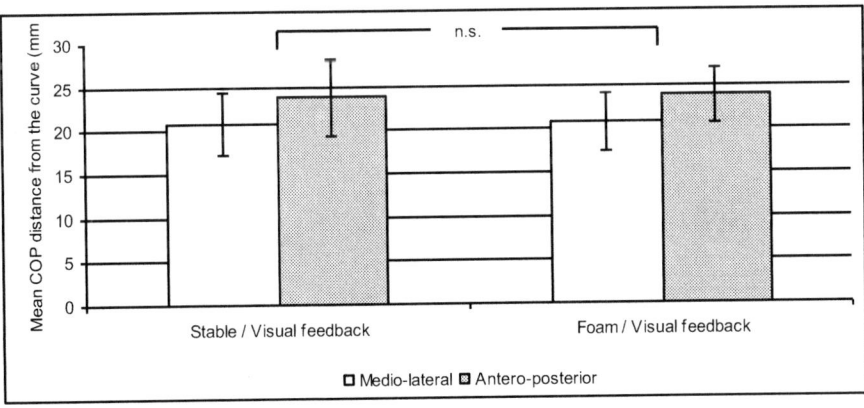

Figure 2. Mean COP distance from the curve in M-L and A-P direction registered during visually-guided COM tracking task while standing on either stable or foam surface.

As has been shown (Potočárová et al., 2009) there are no significant differences in mean COP distance from the curve in antero-posterior and medio-lateral direction while performing visually-guided COM tracking task on stable surface. We were interested whether dynamic conditions would better differentiate sensorimotor parameters in A-P and M-L direction during such a task-oriented sensorimotor exercise. Therefore, we evaluated an accuracy of visual feedback control of COP movement in antero-posterior and medio-lateral direction during visually-guided COM tracking task performed under different stance support conditions.

Results showed (Figure 3) no significant differences in mean COP distance from horizontally and vertically flowing curve while standing on stable and foam surface. However, its values during stance on spring-supported platform were significantly ($p \leq 0.01$) higher in antero-posterior than in medio-lateral direction. A combination of spring-supported platform and foam showed the same tendency but its values were only slightly higher than during standing on spring-supported platform. These differences were caused mainly by increasing the COP distance from horizontally flowing curve. Its values were even significantly ($p \leq 0.01$) higher as compared to those registered during stance on stable and foam surface (Figure 4). It means that **dynamic conditions better differentiate sensorimotor parameters in antero-posterior and medio-lateral direction during visually-guided COM tracking task.**

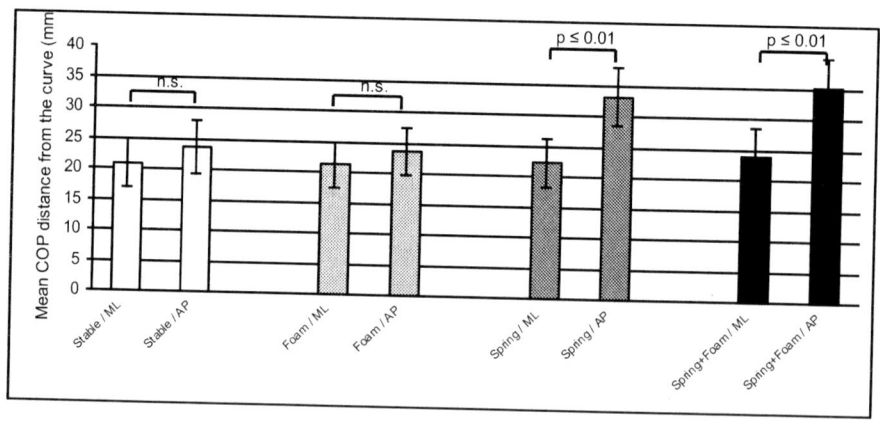

Figure 3. Mean COP distance from the curve in M-L and A-P direction registered during visually-guided COM tracking task under various stance conditions.

These findings may be of importance for the conception and evaluation of visual feedback therapy interventions. For instance, Van Peppen et al. (2006) argued that visual feedback training while bilateral standing on two force plates was not superior to conventional therapy. To provide visual feedback in more demanding and functional balance tasks (e.g., the stance on spring-supported platform) may represent more effective alternative than performing task-oriented sensorimotor exercise on stable surface. However, further studies are needed to prove this assumption.

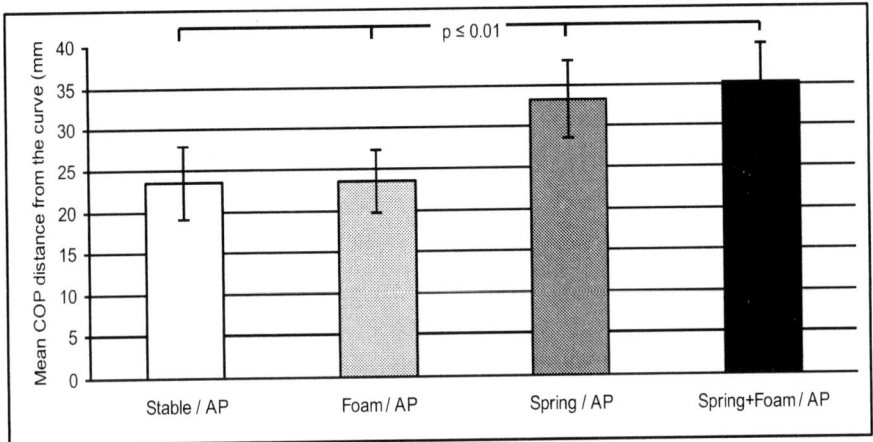

Figure 4. Mean COP distance from horizontally flowing curve registered during visually-guided COM tracking task under various stance conditions.

SENSORIMOTOR EXERCISES: ACUTE ADJUSTMENTS VS. CHRONIC ADAPTATIONS

Experience gained from previous studies served as a basis for designing training programs for various populations. For instance, one study showed that highly-skilled motor behavior in athletes of free-style sports does not contribute to more accurate visual feedback control of COP movement during visually-guided COM tracking task when compared to rowers and cyclists. However, it remains unclear whether development of more precise proprioceptive acuity during task-oriented sensorimotor training contributes to better postural stability or whether enhancement of ability to maintain balance under dynamic conditions after instability agility training improves proprioceptive acuity. In order to partly answer this question we examined the effect of various interventions on sensorimotor parameters (Table 2).

Various groups of subjects volunteered to participate in the studies. All of them were informed on the procedures and on the main purpose of the study. The procedures presented were in accordance with the ethical standards on human experimentation. Information on methods used can be found in related articles.

Table 2. Various training approaches used for improvement of sensorimotor performance

	Proprioceptive stimulation training	Task-oriented sensorimotor training	Instability agility / resistance training
Type of the task	Quiet standing / Performing semi-squats	Active regulation of COM movement	Postural responses to perturbations
Feedback provided	No	Visual	No
Stimuli presentation	No	One	Multiple (e.g., secondary reaction task)
Stance conditions	Static	Static / Dynamic (e.g., spring-supported platform)	Dynamic (e.g., wobble board)
Specific exercise device required	Yes	Yes	No

SERIAL MECHANICAL PROPRIOCEPTIVE STIMULATION

A) Postural Sway Response to Serial Mechanical Proprioceptive Stimulation

This study (Zemková, Hamar, 2008a) evaluated the effect of serial mechanical proprioceptive stimulation of the same frequency and amplitude, however of different durations (15, 60, 180, and 360 seconds, respectively) on parameters of static and dynamic balance.

Proprioceptive stimuli were applied by means of a special strength exercise device producing short-term counter movements (at the frequency of 10 Hz and amplitude of 3 mm eliciting force peaks of 3 g within 3 ms corresponding to the force gradient of 300 N/ms) developed in our department by Hamar (2002-04). Postural stability was evaluated under both static and dynamic conditions (antero-posterior and medio-lateral randomly sliding platform). The COP velocity was registered at 100 Hz by means of the posturography system FiTRO Sway Check based on dynamometric platform.

It has been found that **prolonged proprioceptive stimulation** applied to lower limbs **transiently impairs static balance** (Figure 5), but facilitates **dynamic balance** adjustment leading to its **temporary improvement** (Figure 6). In both cases such effects become more pronounced as duration of stimulation increases.

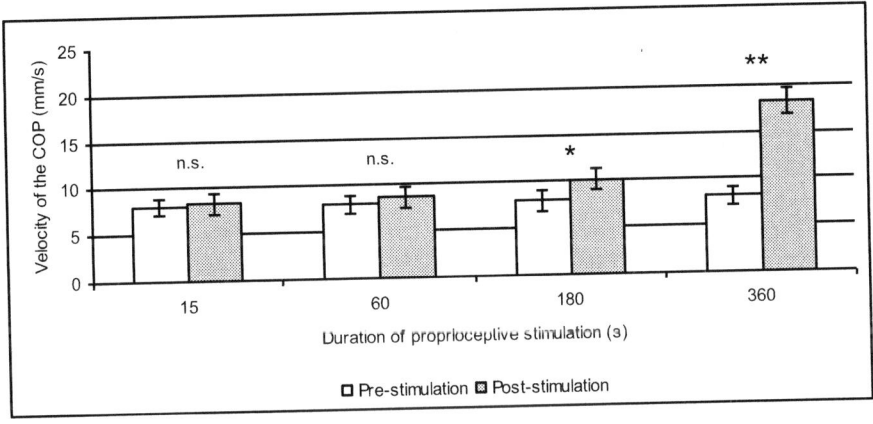

* $p \leq 0.05$, ** $p \leq 0.01$

Figure 5. The COP velocity registered under static conditions prior to and after proprioceptive stimulation of different duration.

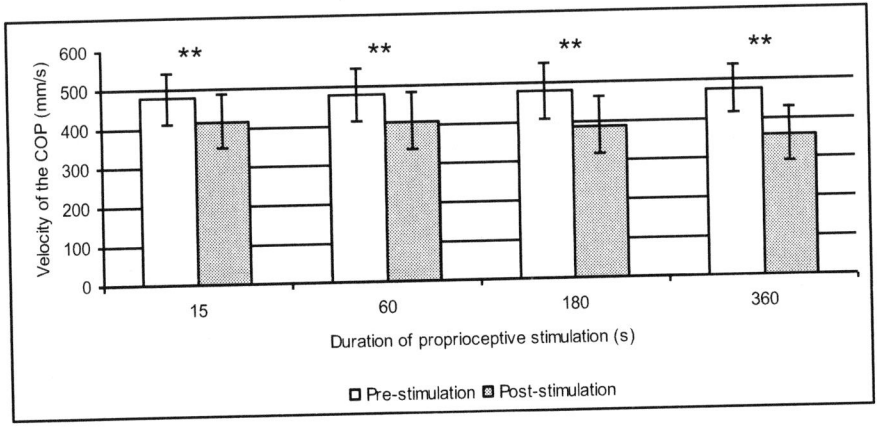

** $p \leq 0.01$

Figure 6. The COP velocity registered under dynamic conditions prior to and after proprioceptive stimulation of different duration.

In another study (Zemková, Hamar, 2007) parameters of balance were compared after lower limb resistance exercise (6 sets of 6 squats with an additional load of 75% of body weight, each session separated by 2 min of rest) performed under normal conditions and under influence of proprioceptive stimulation, respectively. Vertical counter shocks (frequency 10 Hz, amplitude 3 mm) were applied by means of a special device as described above.

Results showed (Figure 7) that squats performed under the influence of proprioceptive stimulation had an early phase of recovery (about 70 seconds) more detrimental effect on parameters of balance than those performed under normal conditions. It means that **additional proprioceptive stimulation enhances an acute effect of lower limbs resistance exercise on parameters of balance**.

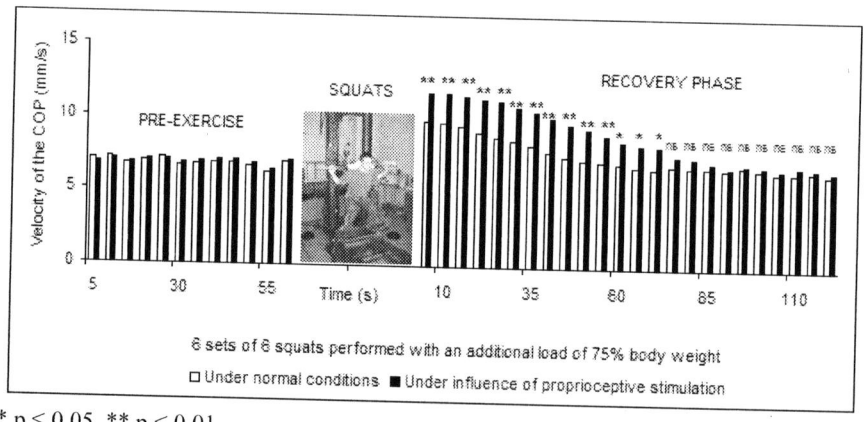

* $p \leq 0.05$, ** $p \leq 0.01$

Figure 7. The COP velocity after squats performed under normal conditions and under influence of proprioceptive stimulation, respectively.

B) The Effect of 3 Months of Serial Mechanical Proprioceptive Stimulation on Neuromuscular Perfomance in Older Women

Findings from previous studies evaluating the acute effect of proprioceptive stimulation of different duration and its combination with resistance exercise on parameters of balance provided an important information for design of following training study. We evaluated the effect of 3 months of proprioceptive stimulation training applied to lower extremities on neuromuscular perfomance in older women.

Subjects underwent (3-times/week) two different forms of exercise, either stood with slightly flexed knees or performed semi-squats on platform producing vertical counter shocks. The intensity of exercise in the first case increased by lengthening the time of stimulation, whereas in the second by additional load. Proprioceptive stimuli were applied by means of a special strength exercise device producing short-term counter movements at the frequency of 10 Hz and amplitude 3 mm as described above.

It has been found that experimental group **improved significantly in agility** (Zemková et al., 2006b), **balance** (Zemková et al., 2007a), and **explosive power of lower limbs** (Zemková, Hamar, 2008b). This effect was more evident when during proprioceptive stimulation the resistance exercise (i.e., semi-squats) was performed. Contrary to this, control group failed to show any significant improvement in these abilities. Such positive changes may be ascribed to the enhancement of neuroregulatory functions, namely increased rate of motoneuron firing and better synchronisation of motor units activation.

These findings indicate that in elderly population the mechanical proprioceptive stimulation applied to lower limbs might enhance neuromuscular performance similarly to resistance training. It may have a practical impact on decrease risk of falling with subsequent reduction of complications affecting namely elderly population.

ACUTE ADJUSTMENTS VS. CHRONIC ADAPTATIONS ASSOCIATED WITH SERIAL MECHANICAL PROPRIOCEPTIVE STIMULATION

Table 3. Acute and training effect of serial mechanical proprioceptive stimulation on COP velocity registered in static conditions

Task	Acute effect on COP velocity	Training effect on COP velocity
Standing on platform producing short-term counter shocks of different duration	↑	↓
Performing semi-squats under influence of proprioceptive stimulation	↑	↓

TASK-ORIENTED SENSORIMOTOR EXERCISES

A) The Effect of Task-Oriented Sensorimotor Exercise on Visual Feedback Control of Body Position and Body Balance

In this study (Zemková, Hamar, 2010b) we evaluated the effect of task-oriented sensorimotor exercise on visual feedback control of body position and parameters of static and dynamic balance. The task of the subjects was to hit the target randomly appearing in one of the corners of the screen by horizontal shifting of COM in appropriate direction while standing on unstable spring-supported platform equipped with PC system for feedback monitoring of COM movement. The test consisted of 20 sets of 60 stimuli with 2 min rest in-between. Time, distance, and velocity of COP trajectory between stimulus appearance and its hit by visually-guided COM movement on the screen were registered by means of the system FiTRO Sway Check developed in our department by Hamar (2007-09).

Results showed (Figure 8 – 10) that response time and distance of sway trajectory between stimulus appearance and its hit by visually-guided COM movement on the screen decreased and sway velocity increased with repeated trials. Such faster responses to visual stimuli may be ascribed to more precise perception of COM position and regulation its movement by horizontal shifting of COM in appropriate direction according to position of stimulus on the screen. However, practice of visually-guided COM target-matching task was not beneficial for improvement of postural stability under static and dynamic conditions (Figure 11 a, b). It means that **task-oriented sensorimotor exercise acutely enhances visual feedback control of body position but not static and dynamic balance** (Table 4).

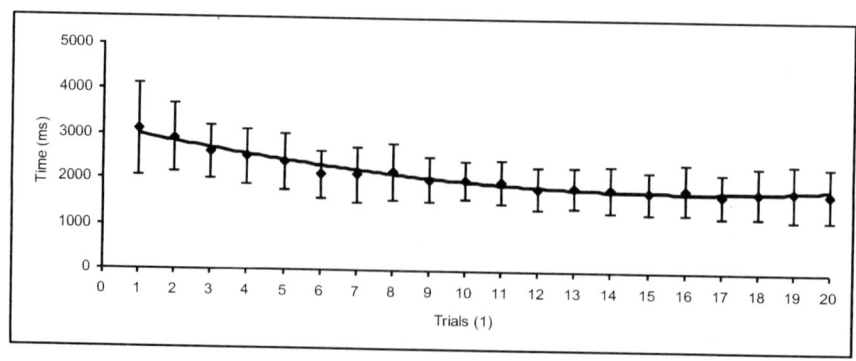

Figure 8. Response time measured during task-oriented sensorimotor exercise .

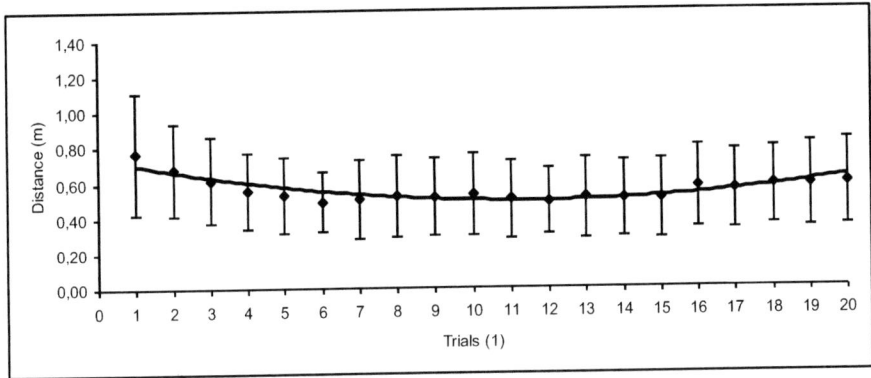

Figure 9. Distance of sway trajectory measured during task-oriented sensorimotor exercise.

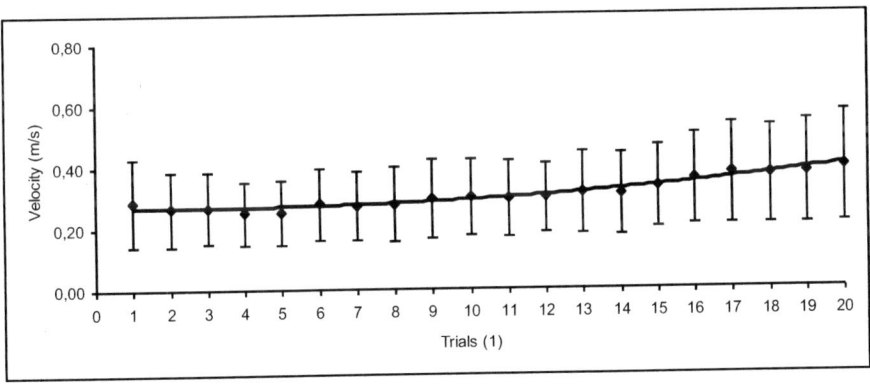

Figure 10. Sway velocity measured during task-oriented sensorimotor exercise.

Table 4. Summary of the results

Test	Parameter	Learning effect
Static balance	COP velocity (mm/s)	–
Dynamic balance	COP velocity (mm/s)	–
Task-oriented sensorimotor exercise	Response time (ms)	↓**
	Distance of sway trajectory (m)	↓*
	Sway velocity (m/s)	↑*

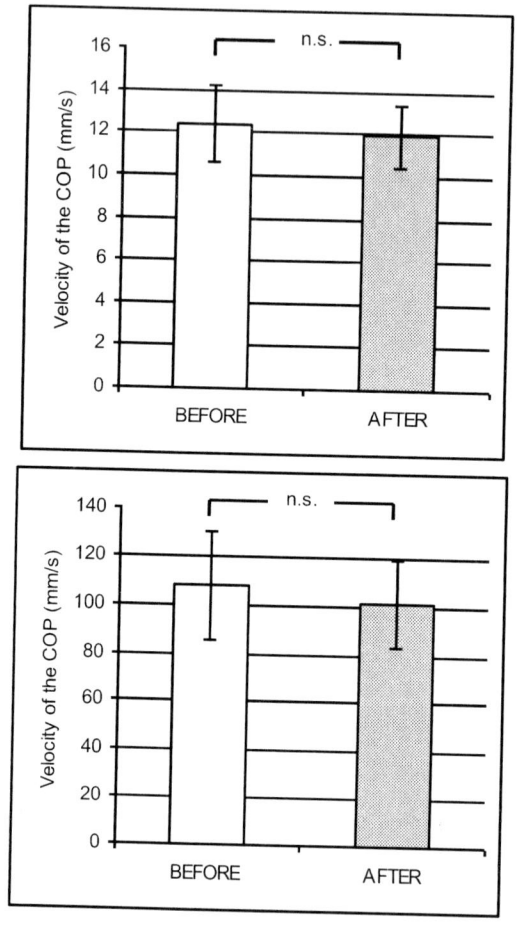

Figure 11. The COP velocity registered in (a) static and (b) dynamic conditions prior to and after 20 sets of task-oriented sensorimotor exercise.

B) The Effect of 3 Weeks of Task-Oriented Sensorimotor Training on Neuromuscular Performance in Untrained Subjects

Previous study showed that task-oriented sensorimotor exercise acutely enhances visual feedback control of body position but not postural stability in static and dynamic conditions. However, question remained whether long-term application of such an exercise would induce changes also in parameters of balance and strength. Therefore, in this study (Zemková, Hamar, 2008c) we evaluated the effect of 3 weeks of task-oriented sensorimotor training on neuromuscular performance in untrained subjects. They underwent 3 times a week the exercise consisting of 3 sets of 200 stimuli with 5 min rest in-between. The task of the subject was to hit, as fast as possible, the target appearing randomly in one of the corners of the screen by horizontal shifting of COM in appropriate direction while standing on unstable spring-supported platform equipped with PC system for feedback monitoring of COM movement.

Prior to and after the training, the time, distance, and velocity of sway trajectory between stimulus appearance and its hit by visually-guided COM movement on the screen were registered by means of the system FiTRO Sway Check as described above. The test consisted of 2 sets of 60 stimuli. In the test subjects had to hit the target by shifting COM in one of the four directions according to position of stimulus on the screen. Postural stability was evaluated under both static and dynamic conditions (wobble board). The COP velocity was registered at 100 Hz by means of the posturography system FiTRO Sway Check based on dynamometric platform. The height of squat and countermovement jumps was calculated from flight time registered by PC-based system FiTRO Jumper. Using the same system also the power in the concentric phase of take off was evaluated during 10-seconds test of maximal jumps. Its calculation is based on contact and flight times measured by the contact mattress with accuracy of 1 ms.

Results showed (Table 5) that response time significantly ($p \leq 0.01$) decreased after the training. Though at the same time distance of sway trajectory also significantly ($p \leq 0.05$) decreased, sway velocity significantly ($p \leq 0.05$) increased. Substantial share of the improvements took place during initial 6 - 8 sessions (about 1 week). Also the ability to maintain balance on unstable platform significantly ($p \leq 0.01$) improved. On the other hand, there were no changes in the COP velocity registered in static conditions. Training program used has also proved to be insufficient to enhance jumping performance expressed as the power in the concentric phase of take off, and height of the squat and countermovement jumps. After the same training control group failed to show any significant improvement in variables evaluated.

It was concluded that **task-oriented sensorimotor exercise applied represents a suitable means for enhancement of neuromuscular performance enabling more rapid postural sway adjustments in altered surface conditions.**

Table 5. Summary of the results

Test	Parameter	Pre-post training changes EG	CG
Static balance	COP velocity (mm/s)	–	–
Dynamic balance	COP velocity (mm/s)	↓**	–
Task-oriented sensorimotor exercise	Response time (ms)	↓**	–
	Distance of sway trajectory (m)	↓*	–
	Sway velocity (m/s)	↑*	–
Squat jump	Height of the jump (cm)	–	–
Countermovement jump	Height of the jump (cm)	–	–
10-seconds jumping test	Power in the concentric phase of take off (W/kg)	–	–

ACUTE ADJUSTMENTS VS. CHRONIC ADAPTATIONS ASSOCIATED WITH TASK-ORIENTED SENSORIMOTOR EXERCISE (VISUALLY-GUIDED COM TARGET-MATCHING TASK)

Table 6. Learning and training effect of task-oriented sensorimotor exercise on selected parameters

Parameters	Learning effect	Training effect
COP velocity registered under static conditions	–	–
COP velocity registered under dynamic conditions	–	↓
Response time and distance of sway trajectory registered during visually-guided COM target-matching task	↓	↓

C) Accuracy of Visual Feedback Control of COP Movement in Antero-Posterior and Medio-Lateral Direction Over Repeated Trials

This study (Zemková, Hamar, 2010c) evaluated the effect of task-oriented sensorimotor exercise on accuracy of visual feedback control of COP movement in antero-posterior (A-P) and medio-lateral (M-L) direction. Subjects were provided by feedback on COM displacement on a computer screen while standing on dynamometric platform. Their task was to trace, by shifting COM, a curve flowing either in vertical or horizontal direction. The test consisted of twenty 30-seconds trials randomly performing in each direction. After its completion, additional 6 trials (one to each direction) were performed every 5 minutes. The deviation of instant COP position from the curve was recorded at 100 Hz by means of the system FiTRO Sway Check developed in our department by Hamar (2007-09).

Results showed (Figure 12) that the distance of sway trajectory from the curve decreased in both antero-posterior and medio-lateral directions when repeatedly performing visually-guided COM tracking task. However, a significant ($p \leq 0.01$) improvement was observed only during initial seven trials. After cessation of practice its values slightly decreased over a period of 10 minutes and then gradually increased toward 30 minute of recovery. Such a temporary improvement of visual feedback control of body position may be due to a) improved the ability to more precise perceive COM position through use the proprioceptors, b) improved the motor ability to perform more accurate body movement, and/or c) improved „proprioceptive memory" with repeated trials. Since tracing randomly flowing curves by visually-guided COM movement on the screen likely eliminate the potential confounding factor of proprioceptive memory, the effect may be ascribed mainly to the improvement of sensorimotor functions. Though it is not possible to separate sensory and motor part of this task, one may expect mainly improvement of proprioceptive acuity with practice. It is beacuse the same receptors share on weight transmission from one to other leg namely during regulation of COM movement in medio-lateral direction (cutaneous and GTO receptors) and discrimination of ankle joint position namely during regulation of COM movement in antero-posterior direction (muscle spindle and cutaneous receptors). However, further studies are needed to prove this assumption.

It was concluded that **task-oriented sensorimotor exercise temporary improves accuracy of visual feedback control of COP movement in both antero-posterior and medio-lateral direction.**

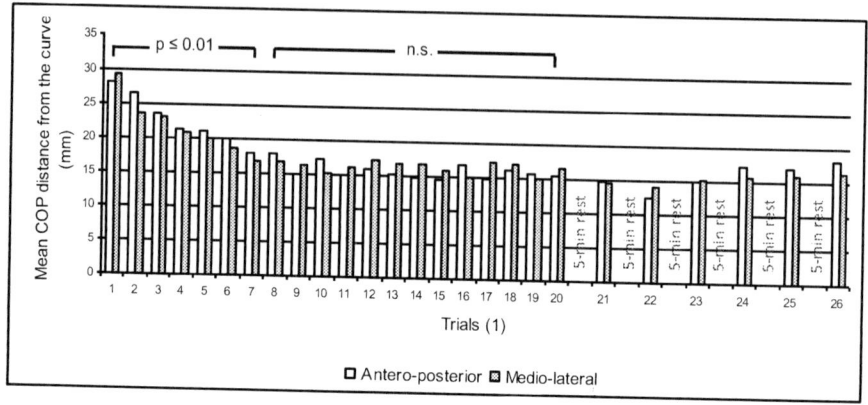

Figure 12. Mean COP distance from horizontally and vertically flowing curve over repeated trials.

In order to evaluate the accuracy of visual feedback control of body position under static and dynamic conditions, we compared mean COP distance from vertically and horizontally flowing curve during visually-guided COM tracking task while standing on stable and unstable surface (wobble board), respectively.

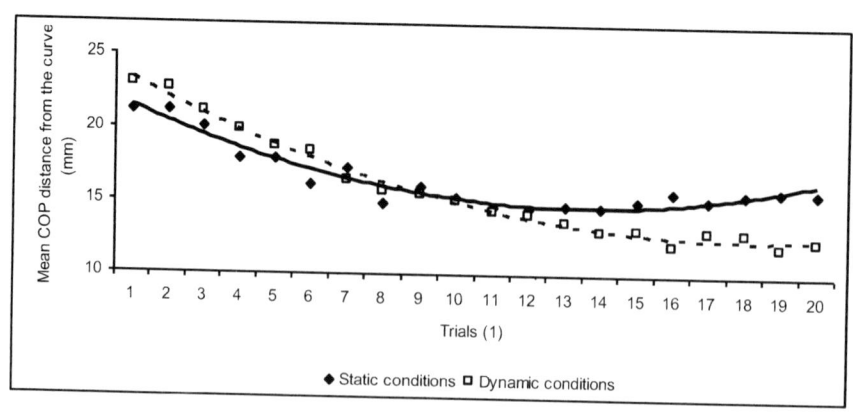

Figure 13. Mean COP distance from the curve registered under static and dynamic conditions, respectively.

Results showed (Figure 13) that the distance of sway trajectory from the curve registered during standing on stable platform decreased from 1st to 8th trial with no further improvement within 20th trial. On the other hand, its values registered under dynamic conditions gradually decreased from the 1st to

20th trial. Consequently, there was greater decline its values over repeated trials (26.3% and 46.1%, respectively). This effect is very probably due to more efficient regulation of COM movement primarily by rotation of ankle joints during stance on unstable platform.

These findings indicate that **learning effect is greater when performing visually-guided COM tracking task under dynamic than under static conditions.**

D) The Effect of 12 Weeks of Conventional and Task-Oriented Sensorimotor Training on Visual Feedback Control of Body Position in Individuals with Functional Disbalances

Previous studies showed that task-oriented sensorimotor exercises improve visual feedback control of body position as well as dynamic balance. However, there is no information whether the same effect may be achieved also by conventional exercise programs consisting of balance exercises. Therefore, we evaluated the effect of 12 weeks of conventional and task-oriented sensorimotor training on visual feedback control of body position in individuals with functional disbalances (Zemková, Hamar, 2010c).

The training during initial four weeks consisted of conventional exercises (4 sessions/week) followed by including visual feedback exercises into the program during next eight weeks (2 of 4 sessions/week). Adaptive changes in sensorimotor parameters were evaluated every week using two different tests. In the first, subjects were provided by feedback on COM displacement on a computer screen while standing on dynamometric platform. Their task was to trace, by shifting COM, a curve flowing either in vertical or horizontal direction. The test consisted of three 30-seconds trials randomly performing in A-P and M-L direction. The deviation of instant COP position from the curve was recorded at 100 Hz by means of the system FiTRO Sway Check. In the second, subjects had to hit the target by horizontal shifting of COM in one of the four directions according to position of stimulus on the screen. The test consisted of 2 sets of 20 stimuli. Time, distance, and velocity of sway trajectory between stimulus appearance and its hit by visually-guided COM movement on the screen were registered by means of the system FiTRO Sway Check based on dynamometric platform. Prior to and after the training also static balance with eyes open and eyes closed was evaluated. The COP velocity was registered at 100 Hz by means of the posturography system, FiTRO Sway Check, based on dynamometric platform.

Results showed (Figure 14) that COP distance from horizontally and vertically flowing curve measured during visually-guided COM tracking task only slightly decreased (8.7%) during initial four weeks. However, its greater decline was observed from the 5th to 8th (10.6%) and from 9th to 12th week of the training (14.5%) when visual feedback exercises were included into the training program.

A similar trend was observed also in case of visually-guided COM target-matching task. However, there were significant individual differences, as shown an example in Figure 15. The subject with good initial performance learned faster as compared to the one with slower response time and longer distance of sway movement registered prior to the training (29.3% and 17.0%, respectively).

Contrary to this, no significant changes in parameters of balance registered in static conditions under and without visual control were found. However, it should be noted that the exercise program led to the enhancement of other regularly measured functional outcomes.

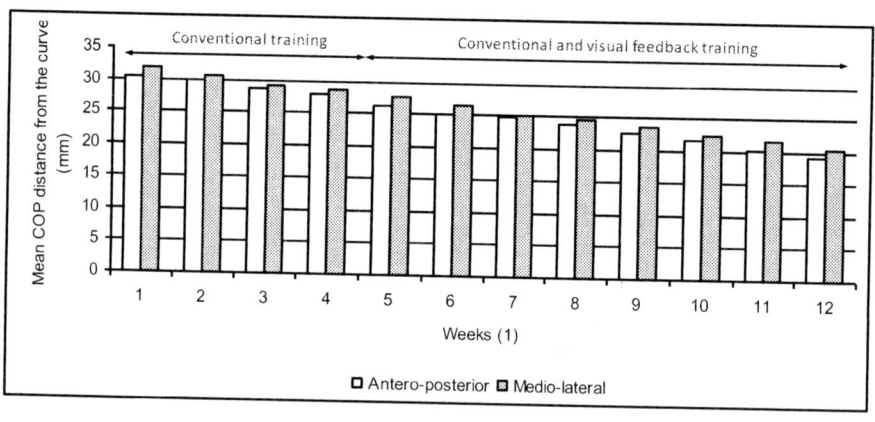

Figure 14. Mean COP distance from horizontally and vertically flowing curve during 12 weeks of different exercise programs.

These findings indicate that **conventional training program** consisting of balance exercises **does not improve visual feedback control of body position**. **Providing visual feedback of COM movement on a computer screen during training contributes to more precise perception of COM position and regulation its movement during different task-oriented sensorimotor exercises.** These findings are in agreement with earlier study of Gibson (1953) who documented that practice with some type of reinforcement (e.g., visual or auditory feedback) results in greater perceptual improvements. Since a limited sample size was used in this study (6 subjects), further investigations are needed to prove the efficiency of exercises based on visual feedback control of body position on sensorimotor performance in individuals with deteriorated coordination due to disease or injury. Also its role in facilitation of learning of other skilled movements should be investigated.

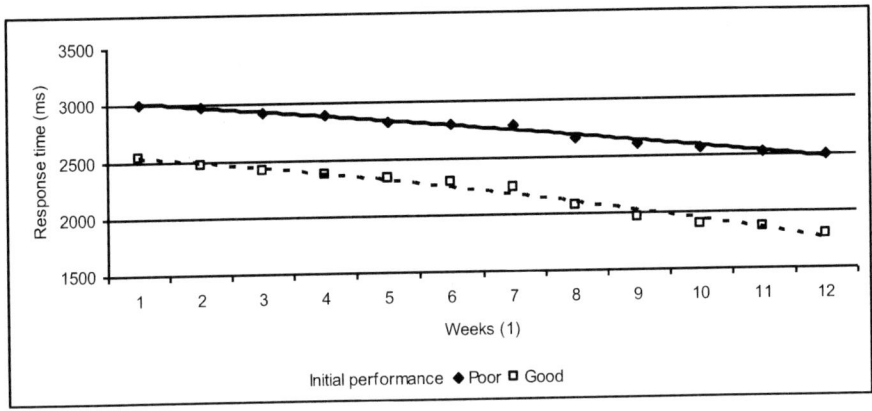

Figure 15. Response time in two individuals with different initial performance level during 12 weeks of exercise program.

ACUTE ADJUSTMENTS VS. CHRONIC ADAPTATIONS ASSOCIATED WITH TASK-ORIENTED SENSORIMOTOR EXERCISE (VISUALLY-GIUDED COM TRACKING TASK)

Table 7. Learning and training effect of conventional and task-oriented sensorimotor exercises on selected parameter

Parameter	Learning effect		Training effect	
	1st-7th trial (visual feedback exercise)	8th-20th trial (visual feedback exercise)	1st-4th week (conventional exercises)	5th-12th week (conventional and visual feedback exercises)
Mean COP distance from both horizontally and vertically flowing curves registered during visually-guided COM tracking task	↓	—	—	↓

COMBINED AGILITY-BALANCE EXERCISES

A) Visual Reaction Time and Sway Velocity While Balancing on a Wobble Board

This study (Zemková et al., 2009b) investigated the reaction time and sway velocity while responding to visual stimuli concurrently with balancing on a wobble board.

A group of PE students responded in random order to either one or two visual stimuli while standing on an unstable support surface for a period of 3 minutes. During the task execution, both sway velocity and reaction time were measured. The COP velocity was registered at 100 Hz by means of the posturography system, FiTRO Sway Check, based on dynamometric platform. Simple and multi-choice reaction times were measured using the FiTRO Reaction Check.

Results showed (Figure 16) no significant changes in simple reaction time while balancing on a wobble board. However, multi-choice reaction time significantly ($p \leq 0.05$) increased from an initial 5-s to the final 5-s period of the test. On the other hand, the COP velocity gradually decreased during a simple reaction task. When responding to two stimuli, there was a significant ($p \leq 0.05$) decrease in COP velocity for an initial 2:15 minutes, which was followed by a slight increase toward the end of the test (Figure 17). Interestingly, multi-choice tasks resulted in greater balance improvement compared to simple reactions.

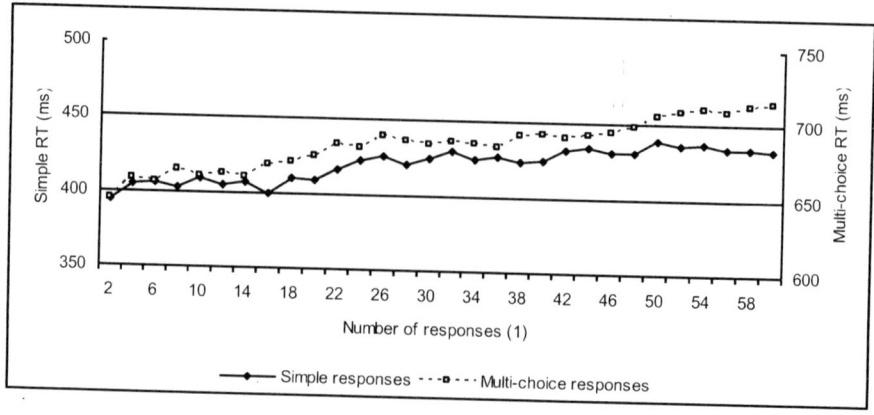

Figure 16. Simple and multi-choice reaction times measured while standing on an unstable support surface.

These findings indicate that **reaction time increases while balancing on an unstable support surface**, whereas **sway velocity declines when concurrently performing reaction tasks**. Having to deal with two tasks at the same time, both of which require controlled processing, can have a different effect on a person's performance depending on the task specificity.

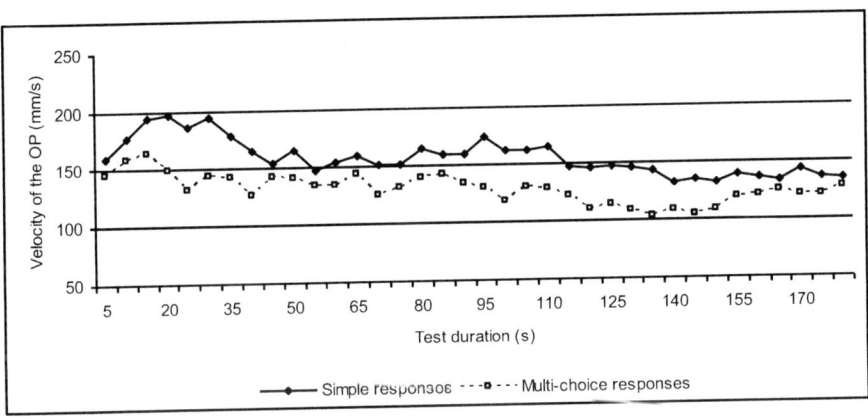

Figure 17. Sway velocity during concurrent RT tasks.

B) The Effect of 8 Weeks of Instability Agility Training on Neuromuscular Performance in Untrained Subjects

In this study (Zemková et al., 2009a) untrained subjects divided into experimental and control groups underwent reaction tasks similar to game-like situations in floorball on wobble boards (one 30 minutes session a week for a period of 8 weeks). Prior to and after the training, sensorimotor parameters, balance and reaction time were evaluated. Sensorimotor parameters including distance, time and velocity of sway trajectory were measured by means of the FiTRO Sway Check, consisting of an unstable spring-supported platform equipped with a PC system for feedback monitoring of COP movement. The task of the subject was to hit, as fast as possible, the target appearing randomly in one of the corners of the screen by horizontal shifting of COM (60 stimuli). Postural stability was assessed under both static and dynamic conditions (wobble board) with eyes open and eyes closed, respectively. The COP velocity was registered at 100 Hz by means of the posturography system, FiTRO Sway Check, based on dynamometric platform. Visual multi-choice reaction time was measured using the FiTRO Reaction Check. Two sets of 20 stimuli were performed in random order, one under normal conditions and another one while balancing on a wobble board. During the task execution both sway velocity and reaction time were measured.

Table 8. Summary of the results

Test	Parameter	Pre-post training changes	
		EG	CG
Bipedal stance on stable platform with eyes open	COP velocity (mm/s)	–	–
Bipedal stance on stable platform with eyes closed	COP velocity (mm/s)	–	–
Bipedal stance on wobble board with eyes open	COP velocity (mm/s)	↓*	–
Bipedal stance on wobble board with eyes closed	COP velocity (mm/s)	/	/
Multi-choice reaction task	Reaction time (ms)	–	–
Responding to visual stimuli concurrently with balancing on wobble board	COP velocity (mm/s)	↓**	–
	Reaction time (ms)	↓*	–
Task-oriented sensorimotor exercise	Response time (ms)	–	–
	Distance of sway trajectory (m)	–	–
	Sway velocity (m/s)	–	–

Results showed (Table 8) that the COP velocity registered under unstable conditions as a parameter of dynamic balance significantly ($p \leq 0.05$) improved. An even more profound decrease ($p \leq 0.01$) in sway velocity was found when responding to visual stimuli concurrently with balancing on a wobble board. Multi-choice reaction time measured under unstable conditions also significantly ($p \leq 0.05$) decreased. However, this effect was not observed while standing on a stable surface. Similarly, there were no changes in the COP velocity registered in static conditions with eyes open and with eyes closed. Unfortunately, no information on changes in dynamic balance without visual control could be obtained because during pre-testing most of the subjects were not able to stand on a wobble board with eyes closed. The training program applied has also proved to be **insufficient to improve sensorimotor performance**. After the same training, the control group failed to show any significant improvement in any of the examined abilities.

It was concluded that balance exercises performed simultaneously with reaction tasks represent an effective means for the **improvement of dynamic balance, namely when responding to visual stimuli**, as well as for reduction of multi-choice reaction time.

ACUTE ADJUSTMENTS VS. CHRONIC ADAPTATIONS ASSOCIATED WITH COMBINED AGILITY-BALANCE EXERCISES

Table 9. Learning and training effect of combined agility-balance exercises on selected parameters

Parameters	Learning effect	Training effect
Reaction time measured while standing on unstable surface	↑	↓
Sway velocity registered in dynamic conditions during concurrent RT tasks	↓	↓

C) The Effect of 6 Weeks of Combined Agility-Balance Training on Neuromuscular Performance in Basketball Players

In this study (Zemková, Hamar, 2010d) elite basketball players randomly divided into experimental (EG) and control groups (CG) underwent a combined agility-balance training (30 minutes in duration) for a period of 6 weeks (4 - 5 sessions/week). Both groups performed reaction tasks similar to game-like situations. However, the EG were performed on wobble boards and the CG on a stable surface. Prior to and after the training, parameters of agility, balance, speed of step initiation, strength differentiation accuracy, and explosive power of lower limbs were evaluated. Postural stability was assessed

Table 10. Summary of the results

Test	Parameter	Pre-post training changes EG	Pre-post training changes CG
Bipedal stance on stable platform with eyes open	COP velocity (mm/s)	–	–
Bipedal stance on stable platform with eyes closed	COP velocity (mm/s)	–	–
Bipedal stance on wobble board with eyes open	COP velocity (mm/s)	↓*	–
Bipedal stance on wobble board with eyes closed	COP velocity (mm/s)	↓*	–
Bipedal stance on wobble board with EO and EC	Rq = EC/EO	↓	–
Simple reaction task	Reaction time (ms)	–	–
Simple agility task	Reaction time (ms)	↓*	–
Multi-choice reaction task	Reaction time (ms)	–	–
Multi-choice agility task	Reaction time (ms)	↓**	–
Step initiation	Max and mean velocity (cm/s)	↑*	–
Estimation of 50% of 1max jump height	Height of the jump (cm)	↓*	–
Drop jump from the height of 45 cm	Contact time (ms)	↓*	–
Countermovement and squat jumps	Δ Jump height (cm)	–	↑*
10-seconds jumping test	Power in the concentric phase of take off (W/kg)	–	↑*

under both static and dynamic conditions (wobble board) with eyes open and eyes closed, respectively. The COP velocity was registered at 100 Hz by means of the posturography system, FiTRO Sway Check, based on dynamometric platform. Using the FiTRO Reaction Check, simple and multi-choice reaction times were measured. The same system was applied to evaluate agility performance, including reaction and movement task. Speed of step initiation was measured using the FiTRO Dyne Premium. Jumping abilities were evaluated by means of the FiTRO Jumper (10-seconds maximal jumps, CMJ, SJ, DJ45). Using the same system, the subject's ability to match 50% of his/her maximal height of the jump was evaluated.

Results showed (Table 10) that combined agility-balance training improved dynamic balance not only under visual control but also in eyes-closed conditions. Training also increased run-out speed that likely contributed to better agility performance, reduced ground contact time during drop jump, and improved the ability to differentiate the force of muscle contraction during repeated jumps. However, such training has been found to be insufficient to improve both simple and multi-choice reaction times and jumping performance. On the other hand, the control group failed to show any significant improvement in examined abilities except for the enhancement of jumping performance (Pact, Δ height of CMJ & SJ).

It was concluded that **balance exercises performed simultaneously with reaction tasks represent an effective means for the improvement of neuromuscular performance in elite athletes**. However, additional exercises have to be implemented into the training program in order to improve reaction time and explosive power of lower limbs.

INSTABILITY RESISTANCE EXERCISES

A) The Short-Term Effect of Different Forms of Resistance Exercise on Postural Sway

Variety of exercises and methods are incorporated into balance training. However, there are no scientific guidelines concerning effective practice schedule for improvement of balance. Therefore, using retention tests we investigated (Zemková, Dzurenková, 2009) a) optimal practice-rest ratios, and b) efficient exercise mode for balance training.

A group of PE students underwent different combinations of practice and rest on two balance tasks, making the percentage of time actually spent in practice (20%, 40%, 60% and 80%, respectively) of the total 30-min period. Thus, the protocol was as follows: a) 6-min practicing (12 x 30-s) / 24-min rest (12 x 2-min), b) 12-min practicing (12 x 1-min) / 18-min rest (12 x 1.5-min), c) 18-min practicing (12 x 1.5-min) / 12-min rest (12 x 1-min), d) 24-min practicing (12 x 2-min) / 6-min rest (12 x 30-s). This schedule was examined under different conditions: a) either balancing or performing squats on wobble board, b) performing squats with different velocities while standing on wobble board, c) performing squats with different additional loads (AL) on wobble board. The learning was tested by administering a transfer test, which was given on the second day. The COP velocity was registered at 100 Hz by means of the posturography system FiTRO Sway Check based on dynamometric platform. While exercising and standing on stabilographic platform, cardiorespiratory parameters were monitored using breath-by-breath system Spiroergometry CS 200. Velocity of movement during squats was measured using the FiTRO Dyne Premium.

Results showed that for balancing on wobble board, the optimal condition for learning occurred when 80% of the time was spent practicing. However, by adding squats, such a combination of 2-min practice and 30-s rest induced a gradual increase in ventilation and heart rate (peak values about 13.4%). Subjects also reported fatigue in lower limbs, which influenced their ability to perform exercise properly. The transfer test showed that for squats performing on wobble board, the optimal condition for learning occurred when 40% of the time was spent practicing. In addition, retention tests of various exercise mode showed (Figure 18) that for improvement of balance are more efficient a) squats performing on wobble board than balancing on unstable surface, b) explosive squats (~180 cm/s) than those performing with slower velocity (~90 cm/s), c) squats on wobble board with lower AL (e.g., 25% of body weight) than those performing with higher AL (50% and 75% of body weight).

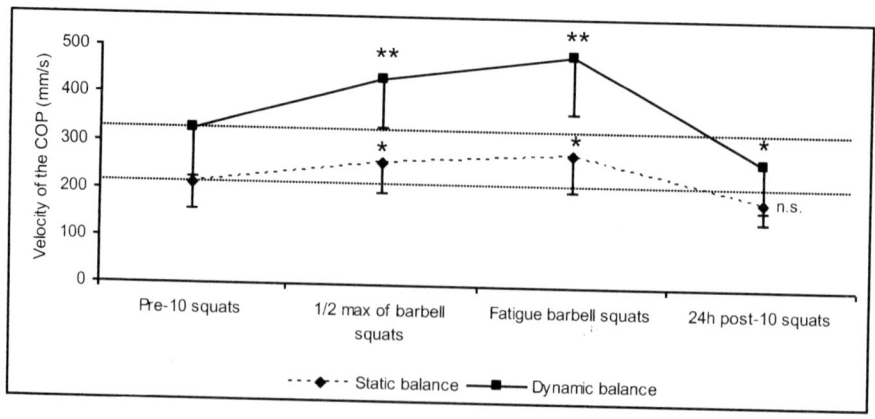

Figure 18. Retention test of static and dynamic balance performed after an interval of one day.

These findings indicate that **explosive squats performing on wobble board with AL of 25% body weight for 1-min with 1.5-min rest in-between (i.e., 12-min practicing / 18-min rest in 30-min session) is effective schedule for improvement of balance**. Previous experience also showed that adaptive changes in balance performance of elite athletes may be induced if such a schedule is provided 4-5 days per week for >25 training days.

B) The Effect of 12 Weeks of Instability Resistance Training on Neuromuscular Performance in Athletes with Previous ACL Injury

In this study (Zemková, Vlašič, 2009) a group of soccer players after ACL reconstruction underwent two months after rehabilitation the combined balance and resistance exercises (e.g., semi-squats, deep squats, wide-stance squats, one-legged squats, barbell squats performed on various unstable support surfaces) in duration of 30 min for a period of 12 weeks (4 - 5 sessions/week). Postural stability was evaluated under both static and dynamic conditions (wobble board and antero-posterior / medio-lateral tilted platforms) during bipedal and one-legged stance. The COP velocity was registered at 100 Hz by means of the posturography system FiTRO Sway Check based on dynamometric platform. Speed of step initiation and the soccer kick was measured using FiTRO Dyne Premium.

Pre-training measurements showed the non-injured-to-injured leg percent differences of 15.7% for static and 24.5% for dynamic balance. Following the training there were no changes in static balance on both legs, on non-injured and injured leg (Table 11). Likewise, the dynamic balance did not change while standing on both legs and on non-injured leg, however a significant improvement on injured leg has been found. In addition, sway velocity significantly decreased during bipedal stance on M-L tilted platform but not on those A-P tilted. Furthermore, run-out speed significantly increased on injured leg but not on non-injured leg. On the other hand, no changes in kick-off speed on injured and non-injured leg have been found.

It was concluded that **resistance exercises performed on unstable surfaces represents an effective means for the improvement of dynamic balance under various conditions and speed of step initiation in athletes after ACL injury**. However more specific exercises should be implemented into the training program in order to improve sport-specific skills like the kick-off speed.

It should be also noted that balance training has been found to enhance rate of force development (Gruber, Gollhofer, 2004; Bruhn et al., 2006; Granacher et al., 2006; Gruber et al., 2007), vertical jump performance (Kean et al., 2006; Taube et al., 2007), and maximal voluntary strength in untrained and impaired subjects (Heitkamp et al., 2001; Hirsch et al., 2003; Bruhn et al., 2006). However, in our study, using explosive power tests in an early phase of post-rehabilitation was limited.

Table 11. Summary of the results

Test	Parameter	Pre-post training changes	
		Non-injured leg	Injured leg
Bipedal stance on stable platform	COP velocity (mm/s)	–	
One-legged stance on stable platform	COP velocity (mm/s)	–	–
Bipedal stance on wobble board	COP velocity (mm/s)		–
One-legged stance on wobble board	COP velocity (mm/s)	–	↓**
Bipedal stance on antero-posterior tilted platform	COP velocity (mm/s)		–
Bipedal stance on medio-lateral tilted platform	COP velocity (mm/s)		↓*
Step initiation	Max and mean velocity (cm/s)	–	↑*
Soccer kick	Max and mean velocity (cm/s)	–	–

CHRONIC ADAPTATIONS ASSOCIATED WITH INSTABILITY AGILITY AND RESISTANCE EXERCISES

Our experience indicates (Table 12) that both instability agility and resistance trainings are efficient to improve dynamic balance, movement velocity and sport-specific performance. However, performing secondary reaction task concurrently with balance exercises can reduce reaction time, whereas force and power development can be achieved by including resistance exercises into the training program.

Table 12. Effects of instability agility and resistance trainings on selected abilities

Abilities	Instability agility training	Instability resistance training
Static balance	−	−
Dynamic balance	↓	↓
Sensorimotor performance	−	−
Agility performance	↑	−
Movement velocity	↑	↑
Jumping performance	−	↑
Sport-specific performance	↑	↑

APPLICATION OF SENSORIMOTOR EXERCISES IN SPORTS TRAINING AND REHABILITATION

Contrary to strength research, scarce reports demonstrate acute adjustments and adaptive changes in parameters of neuromuscular function induced by novel form of interventions like platform feedback exercises. Therefore we intended to partly fill in this gap by investigation the effect of conventional and task-oriented sensorimotor exercises on neuromuscular performance.

It has been found (Table 13) that improvement of more precise perception of COM position and regulation its movement after visual feedback training contributes also to better ability to maintain balance under dynamic conditions. On the other hand, improvement of dynamic balance after instability agility training does not enhance accuracy of visual feedback control of body position. These findings indicate that **task-oriented sensorimotor exercises** represent more effective means for **improvement of both reflexive responses of balance and voluntary movement** than combined agility-balance exercises. However, both exercises were proved to be insufficient to enhance explosive power of lower limbs. For this purpose the instability resistance exercises seems to be more appropriate alternative.

Table 13. Possible effects of balance and visual feedback exercises on balance characteristics

Intervention	Proposed training effects on balance characteristics			
	Static balance	Dynamic balance	Stance symmetry	Accuracy of COM movement
Balance exercises	—	↓	?	—
Visual feedback exercises	—	↓	↑ (when using two force plates)	↑

In summary, for improvement of neuromuscular performance in athletes and healthly subjects, the instability agility and resistance exercises should be applied. On the other hand, for retraining balance function in individuals after injury, using visual feedback exercise seems to be a promising tool that could complement existing rehabilitation methods. It may be of potential use also in elderly populations, for decreasing risk of falling and reduction of health-related consequences.

The comparison of sensorimotor parameters before and after training or rehabilitation may not only provide information on physiological adaptations (e.g., improvement in proprioceptive function) but also on mechanical changes in technique (e.g., more precise regulation of COM movement with less effort). In fact, maximum certainty, minimum energy expenditure, and minimum movement time of goal achievement are three essential features of motor skills proposed by the psychologist E.R. Guthrie (1952). Though several studies investigated the relationship between level of motor skills and proprioceptive acuity, the results often depended on the task in which they were measured. In order to evaluate the effect of novel task-oriented sensorimotor exercises on neuromuscular performance, the methods allowing measurement during functional tasks are needed. This issue is an object of our subsequent study.

ACKNOWLEDGMENT

This project was supported through a Scientific Grant Agency of the Ministry of Education of the Slovak Republic and the Slovak Academy of Sciences (No. 1/0611/08).

REFERENCES

Anderson, K., Behm, D.G. (2005). The impact of instability resistance training on balance and stability. *Sports Med,* 35(1): 43-53.

Barclay-Goddard, R., Stevenson, T., Poluha, W., Moffatt, M.E., Taback, S.P. (2004). Force platform feedback for standing balance training after stroke. *Cochrane Database Syst Rev,* 18(4): CD004129.

Bruhn, S., Kullmann, N., Gollhofer, A. (2006). Combinatory effects of high-intensity-strength training and sensorimotor training on muscle strength. *Int J Sports Med,* 27(5): 401-6.

Buchanan, J.J., Horak, F.B. (1999). Emergence of postural patterns as a function of vision and translation frequency. *J Neurophysiol,* 81: 2325-39.

Gibson, E.J. (1953). Improvement in perceptual judgements as a function of controlled practice or training. *Psychol Bull,* 50(6): 401-31.

Granacher, U., Gollhofer, A., Strass, D. (2006). Training induced adaptations in characteristics of postural reflexes in elderly men. *Gait Posture*, 24: 459-66.

Gruber, M., Gollhofer, A. (2004). Impact of sensorimotor training on the rate of force development and neural activation. *Eur J Appl Physiol*, 92: 98-105.

Gruber, M., Gruber, S.B., Taube, W., Schubert, M., Beck, S.C., Gollhofer, A. (2007). Differential effects of ballistic versus sensorimotor training on rate of force development and neural activation in humans. *J Strength Cond Res*, 21: 274-82.

Guthrie, E.R. (1952). The psychology of learning. New York: Harper & Row.

Hamar, D., Kampmiller, T., Schickhofer, P., Gažovič, O., Zemková, E., Vanderka, M., Pátek, R., Baron, R., Bachl, N., Tchan, H. (2002-04). The effect of serial mechanical proprioceptive stimulation on the parameters of muscle contraction and efficiency of strength training. *The project of the Scientific Grant Agency of the Ministry of Education of the Slovak Republic and the Slovak Academy of Sciences*, No. 1/9192/02.

Hamar, D., Schickhofer, P., Zemková, E., Gažovič, O., Böhmerová, Ľ., Grmanová, K., Pelikánová, J. (2007-09). Nonharmonic proprioceptive stimulation as a means for the enhancement of neuromuscular function. *The project of the Scientific Grant Agency of the Ministry of Education of the Slovak Republic and the Slovak Academy of Sciences*, No. 1/4504/07.

Hamar, D. (2008). Performačné testy stability postoja. *National Congress of Sports Medicine „Aktuálne problémy telovýchovného lekárstva"*. Trenčín: Slovak Society of Sports Medicine, 12-3.

Heitkamp, H.C., Horstmann, T., Mayer, F., Weller, J., Dickhuth, H.H. (2001). Gain in strength and muscular balance after balance training. *Int J Sports Med*, 22: 285-90.

Hirsch, M.A., Toole, T., Maitland, C.G., Rider, R.A. (2003). The effects of balance training and high-intensity resistance training on persons with idiopathic Parkinson's disease. *Arch Phys Med Rehabil*, 84: 1109-17.

Kean, C.O., Behm, D.G., Young, W.B. (2006). Fixed foot balance training increases rectus femoris activation during landing and jump height in recreationally active women. *J Sports Sc Med*, 5: 138-48.

Mergner, T., Schweigart, G., Maurer, C., Blumle, A. (2005). Human postural responses to motion of real and virtual visual environments under different support base conditions. *Exp Brain Res*, 167: 535-56.

Nashner, L.M. (1976). Adapting reflexes controlling the human posture. *Exp Brain Res*, 26: 59-72.

Oddsson, L.I.E., Zemková. E., Dwyer, A., Chow, A., Meyer, P., Wall, C., Bloomberg, J. (2006a). A ground-based research analog for spaceflight effects on gait and balance – Development of evidence-based rehabilitation. *National Space Biomedical Research Institute*

Investigators Retreat. Texas: League City, South Shore Harbour Conference Center.

Oddsson, L.I.E., Bloomberg, J.J., Zemková, E., Dwyer, A., Chow, A., Meyer, P., Wall, C. (2006b). Development of in-flight countermeasures with multimodal effects – Muscle strength and balance function. 7th *Symposium on the role of the vestibular organs in space exploration.* The Netherlands: Noordwijk, ESTEC.

Oddsson, L.I.E., Karlsson, R., Konrad, J., Ince, S., Williams, S.R., Zemková, E. (2007). A rehabilitation tool for functional balance using altered gravity and virtual reality. *J Neuroeng Rehabil,* 4(25): 2-7.

Potočárová, L., Zemková, E., Hamar, D. (2009). Vizuálne spätnoväzobné riadenie pohybu ťažiska v predozadnom a bočnom smere. 3rd *International Students Scientific Confrerence of Kinanthropology „Sport jako životní styl".* Brno: 1-7.

Priplata, A.A., Niemi, J.B., Harry, J.D. et al. (2003). Vibrating insoles and balance control in elderly people. *Lancet,* 362: 1123-4.

Redfern, M.S., Jennings, J.R., Martin, C., Furman, J.M. (2001). Attention influences sensory integration for postural control in older adults. *Gait Posture,* 14(3): 211-6.

Taube, W., Kullmann, N., Leukel, C., Kurz, O., Amtage, F., Gollhofer, A. (2007). Differential reflex adaptations following sensorimotor and strength training in young elite athletes. *Int J Sports Med,* 28: 999-1005.

Taube, W., Leukel, C., Gollhofer, A. (2008). Influence of enhanced visual feedback on postural control and spinal reflex modulation during stance. *Exp Brain Res,* 188(3): 353-61.

Teasdale, N., Bard, C., Larue, J., Fleury, M. (1993). On the cognitive penetrability of postural control. *Exp Aging Res,* 19: 1-13.

Torvinen, S., Kannus, P., Sievänen, H., Järvinen, T.A., Pasanen, M., Kontulainen, S., Järvinen, T.L., Järvinen, M., Oja, P., Vuori, I. (2002). Effect of four-month vertical whole body vibration on performance and balance. *Med Sci Sports Exerc,* 34(9): 1523-8.

Torvinen, S., Kannus, P., Sievänen, H., Järvinen, T.A., Pasanen, M., Kontulainen, S., Nenonen, A., Järvinen, T.L., Paakkala, T., Järvinen, M., Vuori, I. (2003). Effect of 8-month vertical whole body vibration on bone, muscle performance, and body balance: a randomized controlled study. *J Bone Miner Res,* 18(5): 876-84.

Van Peppen, R.P., Kortsmit, M., Lindeman, E., Kwakkel, G. (2006). Effects of visual feedback therapy on postural control in bilateral standing after stroke: a systematic review. *J Rehabil Med,* 38: 3-9.

Verschueren, S.M.P., Roelants, M., Delecluse, CH., Swinnen, S., Vanderschueren, D., Boonen, S. (2004). Effect of 6-month whole body vibration training on hip density, muscle strength, and postural control in

postmenopausal women: a randomised controlled pilot study. *J Bone Miner Res,* 19: 352-9.
Wierzbicka, M.M., Gilhodes, J.C., Roll, J.P. (1998). Vibration-induced postural posteffects. *J Neurophysiol,* 79: 143-50.
Zemková, E., Hamar, D., Böhmerová, Ľ. (2005). The dynamic balance – reliability and methodological issues of novel computerized posturography system. *Med Sport,* 9(2): 76-82.
Zemková, E., Dwyer, A., Chow, A., Oddsson, L.I.E. (2006a). Effects on balance and strength following resistance exercise performed on an unstable surface in a ninety degree tilted environment. *XVI Congress of the International Society of Electrophysiology and Kinesiology.* Torino: 211.
Zemková, E., Hamar, D., Böhmerová, Ľ., Schickhofer, P. (2006b). The effect of 3-month of proprioceptive stimulation on agility skills in elderly women. *Xth International EGREPA Conference „Physical Activity and Successful Aging".* Cologne: 142.
Zemková, E., Hamar, D. (2007). Additional proprioceptive stimulation enhances an acute effect of lower limbs resistance exercise on balance. *International Journal of Applied Sports Sciences,* 19(2): 26-34.
Zemková, E., Hamar, D., Böhmerová, Ľ. (2007a). Effect of three months of serial mechanical proprioceptive stimulation on parameters of balance in older women. *Med Sport,* 11(4): 97-101.
Zemková, E., Oddsson, L.I.E., Dwyer, A., Chow, A. (2007b). The effect of squats performed on an unstable surface in an altered-G environment on strength and balance. *12th Annual Congress of the European College of Sport Science.* Jyväskylä: 346.
Zemková, E., Hamar, D. (2008a). The effect of proprioceptive stimulation of different duration on static and dynamic balance. *International Journal of Applied Sports Sciences,* 20(1): 35-43.
Zemková, E., Hamar, D. (2008b). Proprioceptive stimulation training enhances explosive power in older women. *Acta Facultatis Pedagogicae Nitriensis Universitatis Konstantini Philosophi,* 4(1): 59-66.
Zemková, E., Hamar, D. (2008c). The effect of task-oriented proprioceptive training on parameters of neuromuscular function. *5th International Posture Symposium „Translation of posture mechanisms for rehabilitation".* Smolenice Castle: Slovak Academy of Sciences, 55.
Zemková, E., Dzurenková, D. (2009). Effective practice schedule for improvement of balance. *14th Annual Congress of the European College of Sport Science.* Oslo: 616-7.
Zemková, E., Hamar, D. (2009). Accuracy of visual feedback control of body position during task-oriented sensorimotor exercise in various populations. *Sport Science,* 2(2), 41-46.

Zemková, E., Vlašič, M. (2009). The effect of instability resistance training on neuromuscular performance in athletes after anterior cruciate ligament injury. *Sport Science,* 2(1): 17-23.

Zemková, E., Cepková, A., Potočárová, L., Hamar, D. (2009a). The effect of 8-week instability agility training on sensorimotor performance in untrained subjects. *14th Annual Congress of the European College of Sport Science.* Oslo: 617.

Zemková, E., Miklovič, P., Hamar, D. (2009b). Visual reaction time and sway velocity while balancing on wobble board. *KinSi,* 15(3), 40-47.

Zemková, E., Hamar, D. (2010a). Reliability and sensitivity of the test based on visually-guided COM tracking task. *Acta Fac Educ Comenianae* (in press).

Zemková, E., Hamar, D. (2010b). The effect of task-oriented sensorimotor exercise on visual feedback control of body position and body balance. *Hum Mov,* 2 (in press).

Zemková, E., Hamar, D. (2010c). Task-specific acute and adaptive changes in accuracy of visual feedback control of body position. *Sport SPA,* 7(1) (in press).

Zemková, E., Hamar, D. (2010d). The effect of 6-week of combined agility-balance training on neuromuscular performance in basketball players. *J Sports Med Phys Fitness* (under revision).

Zemková, E., Lipková, J., Hamar, D. (2010). The effects of visual feedback and altered stance support conditions on control of body position during task-oriented sensorimotor exercise in elderly women. *Med Sport* (under revision).

In: Trends in Human Performance Research
Editors: M. Duncan and M. Lyons

ISBN: 978-1-61668-591-1
© 2010 Nova Science Publishers, Inc.

Chapter 9

DIETARY CALCIUM – A POTENTIAL ERGOGENIC AID?

Rehana Jawadwala[*]
University of Central Lancashire, UK

ABSTRACT

Epidemiological data suggest a positive relationship between increased calcium intake and decreased fat and total body mass in healthy people (Barr, 2003; Davies *et al.* 2000). An *in-vitro* model suggesting the role of cyclic Adenosine Monophosphate (cAMP) and phosphodiesterase 3B has been implicated in the relationship between calcium and lipolysis (Xue *et al.*, 2001). This short chapter provides a brief background summarising the research that has led to our current knowledge of the relationship between dietary calcium and energy balance, describe their proposed mechanistic links and discuss the potential merits of calcium as an ergogenic aid in certain sporting conditions. Some of the data presented here spans interventions with varying sources of dietary calcium, from dairy to elemental calcium and studying a vast variety of population demographics in different settings over a range of time

---

[*] Please address correspondence and requests for reprints to
Rehana Jawadwala,
University of Central Lancashire,
Preston, United Kingdom, PR1 2HE
e mail rjawadwala@uclan.ac.uk

periods. Even though animal models and *in-vitro* data suggests a strong relationship between an increase in dietary calcium and a decrease in body weight and/or fat mass; human studies have not supported this *in-vivo*. Experiments in total energy expenditure are vastly inconclusive in supporting the hypothesis of calcium aiding energy expenditure, there seems to be an emerging bank of data favouring the shift in substrates towards increased fat oxidation with higher dietary calcium intakes especially under energy deficit conditions. This may be a potential avenue to explore in a variety of sports in terms of higher fat oxidation aiding glycogen sparing, in addition to a favourable shift in body composition with higher intakes of calcium.

Key words: Calcium, body composition, energy metabolism, fat oxidation, endurance exercise.

INTRODUCTION

The identification of factors that influence energy balance is an important issue in the research field of nutrition. Specific sport populations are concerned with energy balance from a number of perspectives. Maintaining ideal body weight/composition for competitions, making weight in certain sports are some of the primary concerns for athletes. Apart from genetic differences, energy intake and physical activity levels and the macro-nutrient composition of the diet are generally considered as some of the major factors that explain variations in energy balance. However, recent experimental evidence has emphasized that a positive or negative energy balance may happen via the influence of factors that have no *a priori* calorific value. This is the case for calcium intake. An inverse relationship between dietary calcium and body weight was first reported in the 1980s following analysis of a survey database (NHANES1) in a study designed to investigate the relationship between diet and hypertension. Following that, data that established a mechanistic link between calcium intake and energy/fat balance were reported by Zemel *et al* (2001). Based on these epidemiological and *in-vitro* studies there has been a flux in intervention trials in recent years in an effort to establish a link between dietary calcium via dairy and/or supplemental route and energy balance. Most of the studies have looked at vastly different dosages, experimental conditions and outcome measures with mixed results. Part of the confounding issue lies in the fact that it is generally accepted that the uncertainty associated with optimal calcium intakes and requirements exists primarily because the body is able to adapt itself to various levels of dietary intake. Thus, it doesn't seem that the *in-vitro* data can lend itself in a straightforward manner to more physiological dose responses of dietary calcium *in-vivo*. For a detailed and comprehensive analysis of studies in this area the readers are referred to some excellent reviews in the field (Zemel, 2001; 2004; 2005; Schrager, 2005; Barba and Russo, 2006; Huth *et al.*, 2006; Major *et al.*, 2008; Christensen *et al.*, 2009). The purpose of this short chapter is to provide a brief background summarising the research that has lead to our current knowledge of the relationship between dietary calcium and energy balance, describe their proposed mechanistic links and discuss the potential merits of calcium as an ergogenic aid in certain sporting conditions.

PUTATIVE MECHANISTIC THEORIES

It has been shown that a low calcium intake tends to be a marker for a poor diet generally (Barger-Lux *et al.*, 1992). Historically speaking, primitive human diets were calcium rich with calcium to energy ratios two to four times that of modern humans (Eaton and Nelson, 1991). The hormonal response to a low calcium intake is an increase in calcitropic hormones such as Para thyroid hormone (PTH) and a corresponding increase in 1,25 Dihydroxy cholecalciferol ($1,25(OH)_2D_3$) concentrations. Because a low calcium intake would have been tantamount to a low food intake, it may be that human physiology used the PTH and $1,25(OH)_2D_3$ response evoked by a low calcium intake to regulate its energy metabolism and thereby adapt to imminent food shortage (Davies *et al.*, 2000). Today, with the calcium intake disconnected from energy intake, the primitive energy conserving response with a low calcium intake may predispose to weight gain.

The framework for understanding this 'anti-obesity' effect of dietary calcium derives from studies of the mechanism of action of *agouti*, the first obesity gene to be cloned. Obese *agouti* mutant mice (viable yellow, A^{vy}) exhibit increased intracellular calcium in several tissues (Zemel *et al.*, 1995). The increase in intracellular calcium is closely correlated with both the degree of ectopic *agouti* expression and body weight. This correlation has led to several mechanistic links between *agouti*, intracellular calcium and regulatory enzymes in lipid metabolism.

In the forefront of this research is the laboratory of M. Zemel and colleagues. They demonstrated that *agouti* protein stimulates calcium influx and promotes energy storage in human adipocytes by inhibiting lipolysis and stimulating *de novo* lipogenesis (Zemel *et al.*, 2000). When dietary calcium is limited, serum calcium levels fall, stimulating the secretion of PTH, which in addition to increasing calcium release from bone through increased bone resorption and reduced renal calcium loss, also promotes the hydroxylation of 25 Hydroxy Vitamin D ($25(OH)_2D$) to its active form, $1,25(OH)_2D_3$. Both PTH and $1,25(OH)_2D_3$ are implicated in the increase of intracellular calcium (Xue *et al.*, 1998). This has lead to the hypothesis that calcitropic hormones may play a role in adipocyte fat metabolism.

Xue *et al.* (2001) reported the link between increased intracellular calcium and lipogenesis in rat adipose tissue. They suggested that the anti-lipolytic effect of intracellular calcium may be mediated by the activation of phosphodiesterase 3B (PDE-3B) leading to a decrease in cyclic adenosine monophosphate (cAMP) and hormone sensitive lipase (HSL) phosphorylation and consequently inhibition of lipolysis. (See Figure 1.)

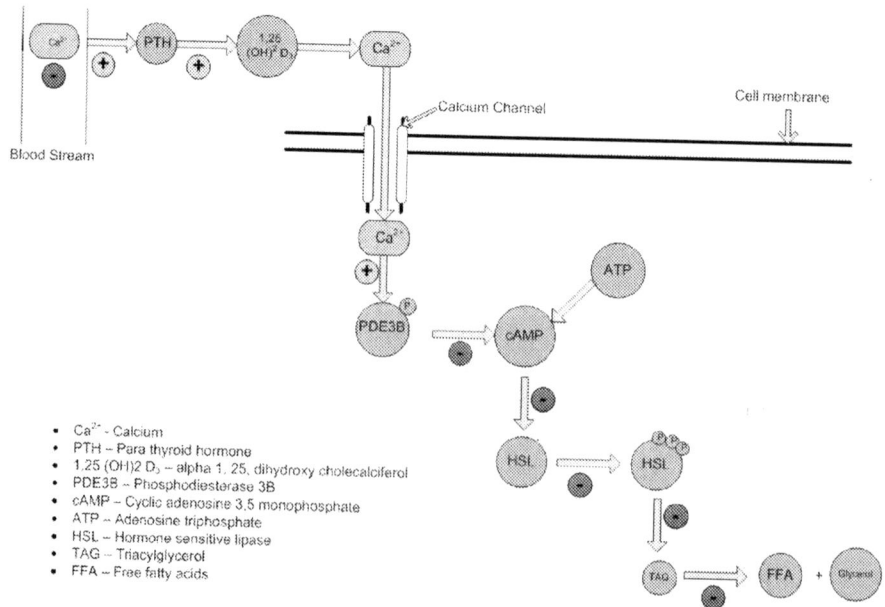

- Ca^{2+} - Calcium
- PTH – Para thyroid hormone
- $1,25(OH)2 D_3$ – alpha 1, 25, dihydroxy cholecalciferol
- PDE3B – Phosphodiesterase 3B
- cAMP – Cyclic adenosine 3,5 monophosphate
- ATP – Adenosine triphosphate
- HSL – Hormone sensitive lipase
- TAG – Triacylglycerol
- FFA – Free fatty acids

Figure 1. Schematic representation of the role of calcium in fat metabolism *in-vitro*.

In addition to the anti-lipolytic role of $1,25(OH)_2D_3$ it may also be involved in the regulation of thermogenesis and energy metabolism in humans. $1,25(OH)_2D_3$ acts via a nuclear Vitamin D receptor (nVDR) to inhibit the expression of uncoupling protein 2 (UCP2) (Shi *et al.*, 2002). UCPs are mitochondrial transporters present in the inner membrane of mitochondria. They have been shown to stimulate mitochondrial proton leak and therefore exhibit a potential role in thermogenesis and energy metabolism (Schrauwen and Hesselink, 2002). Zemel and co workers have reported suppression of 1,25(OH)$_2$D$_3$ by feeding high calcium diets to mice, resulting in increased adipose tissue UCP2 and skeletal muscle UCP3 expression and thereby attenuating the decline in core temperature that would otherwise occur on energy restriction (Zemel *et al.*, 2008). In addition physiological concentrations of 1,25(OH)$_2$D$_3$ seem to have an anti-apoptopic effect on adipocytes, mediated by suppression of UCP2 (Zemel *et al.*, 2008).

Another possible mechanism by which dietary calcium intake might affect adiposity is its effect on the absorption of triacylglycerol from the gastrointestinal tract because of formation of non digestible calcium soaps. Denke *et al.* (1993) reported that calcium fortification (2200 mg elemental calcium/d) increased the percentage of dietary saturated fat excreted in 72 hr faecal collections from 6% to 13% per day. The high calcium diet also significantly reduced total cholesterol by 6%, LDL cholesterol by 13% and apo-lipoprotein B concentrations by 7% when compared to the low calcium diets. In an 85 day dietary intervention trial conducted by Papakonstantinou *et al.* (2003) rats were fed a high calcium diet containing dairy protein or a control diet. Rats on the high calcium diet gained 29% less carcass fat. Welberg *et al.* (1994) studied the effects of calcium supplementation on quantitative and qualitative faecal fat excretion in 24 subjects. They reported a dose dependant increase in fatty acid excretion with supplemental calcium at 0, 2 and 4 g of calcium per day. These studies of calcium's effects on faecal fat excretion predict small effects on total body lipid flux. A person consuming a 2500 kcal/d (~10.5 MJ/d) diet containing one third of energy from fat, taking an additional 2 g elemental calcium/d might be expected to excrete an additional 1% of energy from fat per day and would be anticipated to lose ~3010 kcal/y (~12.6 MJ/y) in stool. This amount of lost energy might explain a change in body weight of ~0.4 kg/y (Parikh and Yanovski, 2003). Thus, these data suggest that faecal fat excretion may only explain a small proportion of the effect calcium seems to have on body weight changes.

The following sections look into detailed research on the effects of calcium supplementation in humans with regards to changes in body weight and composition, energy and substrate metabolism and finally, research in the area of exercise performance benefits.

CALCIUM AND BODY COMPOSITION

Although energy balance is the most critical factor in weight regulation, studies have suggested the calcium supplementation could aid weight loss, in any form of tablet, powder or dairy product. More than 20 years ago a study on the relation between blood pressure and nutrient intake based on data of the 1st National Health and Nutrition Examination Survey (NHANES1) in the USA found a significant inverse association between calcium intake and body weight (McCarron *et al.*, 1984). Similar relationships have also been demonstrated in the Australian population, based on an examination of the data from the National Nutrition Survey 1995 (Soares *et al.*, 2004).

A potential relationship between weight loss and calcium supplementation has been noted in animal studies (Papakonstantinou *et al.*, 2003; Shi *et al.*, 2003; Tordoff *et al.*, 1998; Tordoff, 2001; Zemel, 2000; 2001), large epidemiological studies (Pereira *et al.*, 2002) and human intervention trials (Zemel ,2005b; 2004). But, systematic (Trowman *et al.*, 2006) and non systematic reviews (Barr, 2003) have failed to show a definitive statistically significant correlation between calcium supplementation and weight loss. On the other hand Davies *et al.* (2000) showed a significant negative association between calcium intake and weight for all age groups; on analysing five clinical studies (one intervention and four observational studies). These findings have been confounded by differences in calcium sources, doses, participant demographics, habitual calcium intakes, intervention length and incorporation of exercise and/or caloric restriction. Also the imprecision of the methods of estimating habitual (or baseline) calcium and protein intakes renders estimates of the independent variable inherently uncertain. Methods such as 7-day diet diaries and calcium to protein ratios are less prone to errors as compared to the usual food frequency questionnaires.

A recent meta-analysis of data collected over twelve years from a prospective cohort of men in the United States found that total and dietary calcium intakes were associated with lower weight gain in age-adjusted models in the change analysis. But, they failed to reveal a significant association between dietary calcium intake (dairy or no dairy) with long term weight gain (Rajpathak *et al.*, 2006) with a multivariate model of analysis. This suggests that other diet and lifestyle factors may explain some of the observed changes in the age-adjusted models. Interestingly, the men with the largest increase in total dairy intake gained slightly more weight (3.14 ± 0.11 kg) than did the men who decreased intake the most (2.86 ± 0.11 kg) ($P = 0.03$). This association was primarily due to an increase in high fat dairy intake. These findings have been supported by other studies; Venti *et al.* (2005) were unable to find an association between calcium intake and body size ($r = 0.05$) or adiposity ($r = 0.16$) in Pima Indian adults and children. They hypothesised that part of the reason may be their high fat and high energy diet as observed by Rajpathak *et al.* (2006). These findings from the observational studies have also been substantiated by various controlled randomised trials (Shapses *et al.*, 2006; Thompson *et al.*, 2005; Gunther *et al.*, 2005; Lorenzen *et al.*, 2006) in the recent years.

In addition to the differences in habitual diet related discrepancies, Gunther *et al.* (2005) found contradictory results from two studies from their own laboratory (Lin *et al.*, 2000) examining body mass differences with calcium intervention in healthy normal weight women. Apart from demographical and length of intervention differences they also report that physical fitness of the participants may have a role to play in the different observations in the studies from their laboratory. Even though the physical fitness of the participants in Gunther *et al.* (2005) have been reported as higher compared to Lin *et al.* (2000), where sedentary women with no prior history of physical activity were enrolled on to a 2 year exercise intervention with no supplemental calcium added to their diet (mean reported habitual intake 781 ± 212 mg/d). Interestingly, Lin *et al.* (2000) have reported calcium/Kcal ratios as significant predictors of weight change ($P = 0.01$) and decrease in fat mass ($P = 0.01$) only in women with energy intakes below the noted mean (~1893 ± 373 kcal/d) of their data set. It is therefore possible that not only the physical fitness of the participants but the exercise intervention itself led to some of the reported changes in body composition and influenced the different outcomes of the two studies.

There seems to be two emerging trends in terms of understanding the inconsistency in reported data on the relationship between calcium intake and body compositional changes. Energy balance, high energy/high fat diets and/or exercise protocols seems to have an overriding influence on any small effect that increased dietary calcium may exert via a molecular mechanistic pathway of control of lipid metabolism and/or thermogenesis.

CALCIUM AND ENERGY EXPENDITURE

To explain the inverse relation between dietary calcium and body weight, a few studies have looked at calcium intakes and its effects on 24 hour energy expenditure (EE) (Jacobsen *et al.*, 2005; Bortolotti *et al.*, 2008; Teegarden *et al.*, 2008). But despite increases in fat oxidation in some studies (Melanson *et al.*, 2005; Boon *et al.*, 2005) there does not seem to be much evidence in relation to increase in Total EE (TEE) with an increase in calcium, intake. Jacobsen *et al.* (2005) found that calcium intake had no effect on 24 hour EE or fat oxidation after calcium supplementation (1800 mg/d for 1 week). A similar finding by an earlier study by Melanson *et al.* (2003) found no relation between habitual or acute calcium intakes with 24 hour EE. A recent study by Bortolotti *et al.* (2008) have also reported no increase in resting EE in overweight or obese individuals on a 800 mg/d supplemental calcium for 5 weeks. However, Teegarden *et al.* (2008) reported that overweight women on calorie deficit diets (-500kcal/d) on supplemental calcium (1200 mg/d) for 12 weeks showed an inverse relationship between PTH and TEE and trunk fat mass. But this relationship was not correlated directly to calcium intakes when compared with controls. However, the same study has reported mean serum 25(OH)$_2$ D to positively correlate with a 12-week change in thermic effect of meal (TEM) ($R^2 = 0.17$, $P = 0.04$) independent of group assignment. This is in contrast to the findings by Gunther *et al.* (2005) who have reported a higher TEM after a high calcium (1000-1400 mg/d) intervention compared with a low calcium (<800 mg/d) meal challenge, suggesting a metabolic change in TEM mechanisms.

Some studies looking at surrogate measures of calcium metabolism and its effects on EE and resting metabolic rate (RMR) have also not found any effect on energy metabolism with changes in calcitropic hormone levels. Boon *et al.* (2006) investigated the effect of 7 day oral supplementation of 2000 IU cholecalciferol on energy and substrate metabolism. Although the oral supplementation in combination with low-calcium (352 ± 31 mg/d) and low cholecalciferol (1.6 ± 0.3 mg/d) diet induced significant changes in serum 1,25(OH)$_2$D$_3$ concentrations, no differences in RMR or fat oxidations were observed. These are interesting observations in light that tight regulation of blood calcium levels are maintained through hormonal control of PTH and calcitriol and one of the side effects of calcitriol treatment for hypocalcaemia is weight loss (NIH website). Many of these studies that have looked at TEE or RMR have also looked at fat oxidation changes with calcium supplementation. Some of them (Melanson *et al.*, 2005, Boon *et al.*, 2005) have reported an increase in fat oxidation levels on the same doses of calcium supplementation perhaps suggestive of a shift in substrate partitioning independent of changes in EE.

CALCIUM AND FAT OXIDATION

Based on *in-vitro* studies and epidemiological data, the association between calcium intake and 24-hour fat oxidation in young non-obese humans was first examined by Melanson *et al.* (2003). They examined this association in both self reported habitual calcium intake (mean 1222 ± 116 mg/d) and acute intake (640 ± 44 mg/d). They found a positive correlation and significant between 24-hour fat oxidation and acute calcium intake ($r = 0.38$, $P = 0.03$) but not habitual calcium intake. It is interesting to note that in this study total calcium and not dairy calcium remained significant predictors of 24-hour fat oxidation in backwards stepwise regression models. They have suggested the possibility of a difference in the results between habitual and acute calcium intake on the self-reporting method of calcium estimation. These results have been supported by Cummings *et al.* (2006) who reported that, regardless of the source, calcium intake acutely stimulated postprandial fat oxidation and there was a lesser suppression of free fatty acids (FFA) following calcium rich meals. Thus, it is also possible that some of the effects of calcium on lipid metabolism could be generated rather quickly as $1,25(OH)_2D_3$ has been reported to exert physiological non-genomic effects on calcium metabolism and its putative effects on increasing intracellular calcium (DeLuca, 1998). And indeed in their follow up study Melanson *et al.* (2005) found a ~10% reduction in circulating $1,25(OH)_2D_3$ concentrations but not in plasma calcium, urinary calcium excretion and serum PTH levels. In a study by Boon *et al* (2005) though not as acute as Melanson *et al.* (2003), they also reported a significant difference in change in serum $1,25(OH)_2D_3$ concentrations from 175 ± 16 pmol/L to 138 ± 15 pmol/L in a high dairy/high calcium (1259 ± 9 mg/d ca) group intervention, when compared with a change in serum $1,25(OH)_2D_3$ concentration from 164 ± 13 pmol/L to 198 ± 19 pmol/L in a low dairy/low calcium (349 ± 8 mg/d ca) group in a three 7 day dietary intervention study. Thus, there seems to be a need for further work to study the effects of an acute load of high calcium foods and its effect on fat metabolism via non-genomic actions of $1,25(OH)_2D_3$ or possible other mechanisms.

In terms of long-term interventions, Gunther *et al.* (2005) have studied the effects of chronic high (1000-1400 mg/d) and low (<800 mg/d) dairy calcium intake for one year on 19 healthy normal weight women on their respiratory quotient (RQ) and fat metabolism after a high (> 500 mg) and low dairy calcium (<100 mg) meal challenge, before and after the intervention. The intervention group had a greater decrease in RQ after both the low calcium (-

0.20 ± 0.09 and 0.004 ± 0.08, $P < 0.0001$) and high calcium (-0.12 ± 0.09 and -0.06 ± 0.08, $P < 0.006$) meal challenges. They also reported a corresponding increase in fat oxidation in the intervention group as compared to the controls after both, the low calcium (0.10 ± 0.05 and 0.005 ± 0.04 g/min, $P < 0.0001$) and high calcium (0.06 ± 0.05 and 0.03 ± 0.04 g/min, $P < 0.009$) meal challenges. These results suggest that chronic increased dietary calcium results in the long term adjustment in the ability to oxidise fats and utilise calories, even without high calcium content in the meal. This however, contradicts the findings of Melanson et al. (2003) who have reported no significant changes in fat oxidation rates with a high self reported habitual calcium intake (mean 1222 ± 116 mg/d). Gunther et al. (2005) have not looked at serum $1,25(OH)_2D_3$ concentrations, however they have reported no significant changes in serum log PTH for the control group (0.18 ± 0.62) as compared to the intervention group (0.07 ± 0.49) after one year of the intervention, nor any significant correlations with fat oxidation even when corrected for changes in body composition. But they have reported a negative partial correlation between the 1 year change in log PTH and 1 year change in whole body fat oxidation in response to a high calcium meal but not a low calcium meal. This probably suggests that the homeostatic concentration of PTH suppression may be modified by the chronic intake of calcium.

If the increase in calcium intake is then combined with a caloric restriction then the effects on fat oxidation rates seem to get more pronounced. In a follow-up dairy intervention study by Melanson et al. (2005) the authors found that under energy balance conditions there was no effect of low-dairy (LD) (~500 mg calcium/d/7days) or high-dairy (HD) (~1400 mg calcium/d for 7 days) treatment on respiratory quotient (RQ) or 24-hour macronutrient oxidation. However, under energy deficit (-600 kcal/d) conditions, 24-hour fat oxidation was significantly increased on high dairy diet (HD = 136 ± 13 g/d, LD = 106 ± 7 g/d, $P = 0.02$). One important distinction between the energy balance and the energy deficit interventions was that energy deficit was achieved via a combination of calorie restriction (~100 kcal) and exercise (~400 kcal from an exercise with workload of $70\% VO_{2peak}$). Fat oxidation did not differ between HD and LD in energy deficit conditions when the participants were resting, but only increased during the exercise session and during another two 10 min stepping bouts (96, 72, 96 steps/min). The authors have thus suggested that the increase in fat oxidation rates and decrease in RQ during the energy deficit trials could be due to exercise rather than calcium. However, the energy balance trials also included the step bouts without any difference in fat oxidation rates between the two dietary conditions. This could lead to a possible effect of increased lipolytic effect via increase in dietary calcium intakes under energy deficit conditions but not energy balance conditions. This increase in availability of FFA during exercise conditions could then translate to a higher fat oxidation rate but not in resting conditions where the available FFA in the blood could be re-esterified due to lower energy demands at the time. Another study on high (~1700-1800 mg/d) and low (~475 mg/d) calcium for 7 days by Jacobson et al (2005) found a small but non-significant increase in fat oxidation with a high calcium + normal protein diet (11.5 ± 8 E%) but not with high calcium + high protein diet (7.9 ± 6 E%) when compared to low calcium + normal protein diet (7.4 ± 9 E%). This was matched with a small but non-significant increase in FFA after the high calcium + normal protein diet (66 ± 212 µmol/L) as compared to a non-significant decrease (-117 ± 235 µmol/L) in participants who were on a low calcium + normal protein diet and the ones on a high calcium + high protein diet (-17.5 ± 151 µmol/L). However, unlike the study by Melanson et al. (2005) there was no specific exercise provision in this study. Only spontaneous activity was measured via microwave radar detectors and accounted for as part of the 24-hour EE. Thus, considering the FFA data, in light of the fat oxidation data, it seems to lend itself to the explanation that the increased availability of FFA with increased calcium intakes could be an important factor in determining the increased rates of fat oxidation without any change to TEE. Boon et al. (2005) with a similar research of randomised crossover design with isocaloric diets of high calcium/high dairy (1259 ± 9 mg/d), high calcium/low dairy (1259 ± 9 mg/d) and low calcium/low dairy (349 ± 8 mg/d) have also reported very modest non significant increase in fat oxidation rates (108 ± 7 g/d) following high dairy/high calcium diets as compared with low dairy/low calcium group (100 ± 6 g/d). Considering that most studies have reported very modest changes in fat oxidation rates and it seems that the relation between calcium intakes and substrate metabolism may be more interrelated with lipolysis than oxidation of fatty acids at least in sedentary participants over a 24 hour period. This is evident with observed significant changes in circulating $1,25(OH)_2D_3$ concentrations which has a direct impact on increasing intracellular calcium levels at least *in-vitro* and in animal studies affecting lipolytic and lipogenic hormonal milieu as reported by numerous studies (Shi *et al.*, 2001; Xue *et al.*, 2000; 2001). It is possible that these effects may not reflect normal physiological situations. Another reason for these studies to have reported small but not significant changes in fat oxidation may be due to low statistical power in most human intervention studies described above. Most of these studies have reported studying between

7-20 participants. Boon *et al.* (2005) have stated that from a post hoc power analysis, it was calculated that to reach significant differences in substrate metabolism with the variances and differences observed between groups, the required number of participants would at least be 43 in their study. Thus the relation between fat oxidation rates and calcium intakes in humans requires more in-depth examination particularly the impact of lipolytic mechanisms on substrate metabolism *in-vivo* as that might provide some understanding of the role of calcium in its influence on body composition as seen consistently from epidemiological (McCarron *et al.*, 1984; Zemel *et al.*, 2000; Pereira *et al.*, 2002) and meta analytical (Davies *et al.*, 2000) data.

CALCIUM AND EXERCISE PERFORMANCE

Most data on calcium homeostasis in the blood during exercise is derived from studies examining bone health and exercise. There are not many specific studies exploring calcium intakes and its relation to substrate metabolism during exercise. White *et al.* (2006) reported no significant treatment effect of acute calcium (500 mg) intervention on endurance trained female runners. On a 90 min glycogen depletion trial followed by a 10K time trial performance, the researchers found no difference in fat oxidation rates of appearance of glycerol in the blood stream nor changes in respiratory exchange ratios during the performance test. Acute calcium intake also did not seem to have any influence on time to finish on the 10 K time trial. However, unpublished data from our laboratory (Jawadwala *et al.*, unpublished) has shown that calcium supplementation of 1000 mg/d for 4 weeks had a significant effect on time to finish a 25 mile cycle ergometer time trial (-1.25 ± 0.32 mins, $P = 0.04$) before and after the intervention with highly trained endurance trained cyclists. It is possible that these differences in data may be due to the intervention period. Melanson *et al.* (2005) used a 70% VO_{2peak} protocol in their 7 day high and low dairy intervention study to achieve a ~400 Kcal energy deficit. They found a significant increase in 24 hour fat oxidation rates when their participants were on the exercise protocol between high dairy (HD~1400 mg/d) and low dairy (LD~500 mg/d) groups (HD = 136 ± 13 g/d, LD = 106 ± 13 g/d; $P = 0.02$). They have not looked at any performance measures and perhaps it would be speculative to infer that the increase in fat oxidation rates would translate into glycogen sparing action and thus would have improved performance in this experiment, especially since this population were untrained individuals. However, even with a 4 week intervention of supplemental calcium our data (Jawadwala et al., unpublished) does not support any substantial increase in FFA availability in the blood during the 25 mile time trial or any significant changes in total energy expenditure during the time trial. The main role of lipid mobilisation during exercise is played by β-adrenoreceptor-mediated activation of hormone sensitive lipase in the adipocytes (Holloszy et al., 1998). And since Xue et al. (2001) have demonstrated that intracellular calcium activates phosphodiesterase 3B reducing the intracellular pool of cAMP and thereby suppressing the phosphorylation of HSL, there seems to be merit in a high calcium diet and its purported effects on increased availability of FFA, which in turn should increase fat oxidation during endurance exercise. There are no studies that have looked at ionised calcium in blood in relation to exercise with a calcium supplementation intervention, either acute or chronic. Men'shikov, (2004) have reported an increased availability of FFA with a corresponding decrease in plasma ionised calcium after exercise in trained athletes as compared to untrained controls when performing a endurance cycle ergometer test of 90 min duration (17 kg-m.min^{-1}.kg^{-1}) without any calcium related intervention however. In addition, they reported a multiple correlation between post-exercise plasma FFA, ionised calcium and oxygen consumption in athletes ($r = 0.72$; $P < 0.05$) suggesting an involvement of calcium in FFA metabolism.

Another possible avenue for performance enhancement via the aid of calcium supplementation could be due to the changes in body composition over a period of time. We have observed (Jawadwala et al., unpublished) a significant increase in gross efficiency rates of 25 mile cycling time trial after 4 weeks of calcium supplementation (1000 mg/d) (2.23% ± 1.16%, $P = 0.0001$) and a corresponding increase in economy (7.79 W/L ± 4.06 W/L, $P = 0.0001$). These significant changes in performance parameters corresponded with a small shift in body composition towards lower fat mass (-0.81% ± 0.18%) and concurrent increase in lean mass (0.81% ± 0.18%) of the cyclists ($n = 10$) over the 4 week period with mean total body weight remaining the same. Thus even though there does not seem to be a direct effect of acute calcium load on performance parameters, the influence of calcium on body composition may still be an avenue for further research with respect to its ergogenic properties.

Summary

Calcium plays a variety of roles in the human metabolism and *in-vitro* and animal studies have suggested a strong correlation between increased intracellular calcium and fat metabolism with a concurrent chronic effect on body weight and composition. However, studies conducted in humans are inconclusive towards supporting those data. With calcium levels being very tightly regulated in the body any intervention designed to study its specific role in energy metabolism has obvious challenges in terms of methodology and control of confounding factors. Over and above differences in the source of calcium including dairy and supplemental forms; the measurement of energy expenditure in free living organisms especially in simulated laboratory conditions all further complicate the comparison of different experimental conditions. As we have seen from the evidence presented that even though experiments in total energy expenditure are vastly inconclusive in supporting the hypothesis of calcium aiding EE, there seems to be an emerging bank of data favouring the shift in substrates towards increased fat oxidation with higher dietary calcium intakes especially under energy deficit conditions.

Some future work studying the differences in the shift of substrates during exercise with relation to training adaptations in athletes would enhance our understanding in the area immensely. Trained athletes are better able to utilise fat as a source of energy during sub-maximal exercise (Holloszy and Coyle 1984). If dietary calcium plays a role in lipolysis and thus increasing the availability of FFA, it may aid in increased fat oxidation rates during a given exercise bout. This in turn may help spare glycogen, leading to performance enhancement and/or delay in fatigue. These metabolic shifts may in turn shift the athlete's body composition favourably.

Thus, the potential benefits of understanding the complex role of calcium in energy metabolism span from interventions to ameliorate the spread of obesity, hypertension, diabetes and the other axes of the metabolic syndrome to a potential ergogenic effect on performance.

References

Barba, G. & Russo, P. (2006). Dairy foods, dietary calcium and obesity: A short review of the evidence. *Nutrition, Metabolism and Cardiovascular Diseases*, 16, 6, 445-451.

Barger-Lux, M.J., Heaney, R.P., Packard, P.T., Lappe, J.M., & Recker, R.R. (1992). Nutritional Correlates to low calcium intake (Abstract). *Clinical Applied Nutrition*, 2, 39-44.

Barr, S.I. (2003) Increased Dairy Product or Calcium Intake: Is Body Weight or Composition Affected in Humans? *Journal of Nutrition*, 133, 245S-248.

Boon, N., Hul, G.B.J., Sicard, A., Kole, E., Van Den Berg, E.R., Viguerie, N., Langin, D., & Saris, W.H.M. (2006). The Effects of Increasing Serum Calcitriol on Energy and Fat Metabolism and Gene Expression. *Obesity*, 14, 1739-1746.

Boon, N., Hul, G.B., Viguerie, N., Sicard, A., Langin, D., & Saris, W.H. (2005) Effects of 3 diets with various calcium contents on 24-h energy expenditure, fat oxidation, and adipose tissue message RNA expression of lipid metabolism-related proteins. *American Journal of Clinical Nutrition*, 82, 1244-1252.

Bortolotti, M., Rudelle, S., Schneiter, P., Vidal, H., Loizon, E., Tappy, L., & Acheson, K.J. (2008). Dairy calcium supplementation in overweight or obese persons: its effect on markers of fat metabolism. *American Journal of Clinical Nutrition*, 88, 877-885.

Cummings, N.K., James, A.P., & Soares, M.J. (2006). The acute effects of different sources of dietary calcium on postprandial energy metabolism. *British Journal of Nutrition*, 96, 138-144.

Davies, K.M., Heaney, R.P., Recker, R.R., Lappe, J.M., Barger-Lux, M.J., Rafferty, K., & Hinders, S. (2000) Calcium Intake and Body Weight", *Journal of Clinical Endocrinology Metabolism*. 85, 4635-4638.

DeLuca, H.F. & Cantorna, M.T. (2001). Vitamin D: its role and uses in immunology. *The FASEB Journal*, 15, 2579-2585.

Denke, M.A., Fox, M.M., & Schulte, M.C. (1993). Short-term dietary calcium fortification increases faecal saturated fat content and reduces serum lipids in men. *Journal of Nutrition,* 123, 1047–1053.

Eaton, S.B. & Nelson, D.A. (1991). Calcium in evolutionary perspective. *American Journal of Clinical Nutrition*, 54, 281S-287.

Gunther, C.W., Legowski, P.A., Lyle, R.M., Weaver, C.M., Mccabe, L.D., Mccabe, G.P., Peacock, M., & Teegarden, D. (2006) Parathyroid hormone is associated with decreased fat mass in young healthy women. *International Journal of Obesity*, 30, 94-99.

Gunther, C.W., Lyle, R.M., Legowski, P.A., James, J.M., McCabe, L.D., McCabe, G.P., Peacock, M., & Teegarden, D. (2005) Fat oxidation and its relation to serum parathyroid hormone in young women enrolled in a 1-y dairy calcium intervention. *American Journal of Clinical Nutrition*, 82, 1228-1234.

Holloszy, J.O. & Coyle, E.F. (1984) Adaptations of skeletal muscle to endurance exercise and their metabolic consequences. *Journal of Applied Physiology*, 56, 831-839.

Horowitz, J.F. & Klein, S. (2000). Lipid metabolism during endurance exercise. *American Journal of Clinical Nutrition*, 72, 558S-563.

Huth, P.J., DiRienzo, D.B., & Miller, G.D. (2006). Major Scientific Advances with Dairy Foods in Nutrition and Health. *Journal of Dairy Science*, 89, 1207-1221.

Jacobsen, R., Lorenzen, J.K., Toubro, S., Krog-Mikkelsen, I., & Astrup, A. (2005) Effect of short-term high dietary calcium intake on 24-h energy expenditure, fat oxidation, and fecal fat excretion. *International Journal of Obesity and Related Metabolic Disorders*, 29, 292-301.

Lin, Y.C., Lyle, R.M., McCabe, L.D., McCabe, G.P., Weaver, C.M., & Teegarden, D. (2000) Dairy Calcium is Related to Changes in Body Composition during a Two-Year Exercise Intervention in Young Women. *Journal of the American College of Nutrition*, 19, 754-760.

Major, G. C., Chaput, J.P., Ledaux, M., St-Pierre, S., Anderson, G.H., Zemel, M.B. & Tremblay, A. (2008) Recent developments in calcium related obesity research. *Obesity Reviews*, 9, 428-445.

McCarron, D.A., Morris, C.D., Henry, H.J., & Stanton, J.L. (1984) Blood pressure and nutrient intake in the United States. *Science*, 224, 1392-1398.

Melanson, E.L., Sharp, T.A., Schneider, J., Donahoo, W.T., Grunwald, G.K., & Hill, J.O. (2003). Relation between calcium intake and fat oxidation in adult humans. *International Journal of Obesity and Related Metabolic Disorders*, 27, 196-203.

Melanson, E.L., Donahoo, W.T., Dong, F., Ida, T., & Zemel, M.B. (2005) Effect of Low- and High-Calcium Dairy-Based Diets on Macronutrient Oxidation in Humans. *Obesity*, 13, 2102-2112.

Men'shikov, I.V. (2004). Free Fatty Acids and Ca^{2+} in Blood Plasma of Endurance-Trained Athletes after Prolonged Physical Exercise. *Human Physiology*, 30, 485-489.

Papakonstantinou, E., Flatt, W.P., Huth, P.J., & Harris, R.B.S. (2003). High Dietary Calcium Reduces Body Fat Content, Digestibility of Fat, and Serum Vitamin D in Rats. *Obesity Research*, 11, 387-394.

Parikh, S.J. & Yanovski, J.A. (2003). Calcium intake and adiposity. *American Journal of Clinical Nutrition*, 77, 281-287.

Pereira, M.A., Jacobs, D.R., Jr., Van Horn, L., Slattery, M.L., Kartashov, A.I., & Ludwig, D.S. (2002). Dairy Consumption, Obesity, and the Insulin Resistance Syndrome in Young Adults: The CARDIA Study. *The Journal of the American Medical Association*, 287, 2081-2089.

Rajpathak, S.N., Rimm, E.B., Rosner, B., Willet, W.C., & Hu, F.B. (2006). Calcium and dairy intakes in relation to long term weight gain in US men. *American Journal of Clinical Nutrition*, 83, 559-566.

Schrager, S. (2005). Dietary Calcium Intake and Obesity. *The Journal of the American Board of Family Practice*, 18, 205-210.

Schrauwen, P., & Hesselink, M. (2002). UCP2 and UCP3 in muscle controlling metabolism. *The Journal of Experimental Biology*, 205, 2275-2285.

Shapses, S.A., Heshka, S., & Heymsfield, S.B. (2004). Effect of Calcium Supplementation on Weight and Fat Loss in Women. *Journal of Clinical Endocrinology Metabolism*, 89, 632-637.

Shi, H., DiRienzo, D., & Zemel, M.B. (2001). Effects of dietary calcium on adipocyte lipid metabolism and body weight regulation in energy restricted aP2-agouti transgenic mice. *FASEB J*, 15, 291–293.

Shi, H., Norman, A.W., Okamura, W.H., Sen, A., & Zemel, M.B. (2001b). 1a,25-Dihydroxyvitamin D3 modulates human adipocyte metabolism via nongenomic action. *The FASEB Journal*, 01-0584.

Soares, M.J., Ping-Delfos, W.C., James, A.P. & Cummings, N.K. (2004) Dairy calcium and vitamin D stimulate postprandial thermogenesis: effect of sequential meals. (Abstract). *Asia Pacific Journal of Clinical Nutrition*, 13, S56.

Teegarden, D., White, K.M., Lyle, R.M., Zemel, M.B., Van Loan, M.D., Matkovic, V., Craig, B.A., & Schoeller, D.A. (2008). Calcium and Dairy Product Modulation of Lipid Utilization and Energy Expenditure. *Obesity*, 16, 1566-1572.

Thompson, W.G., Rostad Holdman, N., Janzow, D.J., Slezak, J.M., Morris, K.L., & Zemel, M.B. (2005). Effect of Energy-Reduced Diets High in Dairy Products and Fiber on Weight Loss in Obese Adults. *Obesity*, 13, 1344-1353.

Tordoff, M.G. (2001). Calcium: Taste, Intake, and Appetite. *Physiological Reviews*, 81, 1567-1597.

Tordoff, M.G., Hughes, R.L., & Pilchak, D.M. (1998). Calcium intake by rats: influence of parathyroid hormone, calcitonin, and 1,25-dihydroxyvitamin D. *AJP - Regulatory, Integrative and Comparative Physiology*, 274, R214-R231.

Trowman, R., Dumville, J.C., Hahn, S., & Torgerson, D.J. (2006). A systematic review of the effects of calcium supplementation on body weight. *British Journal of Nutrition*, 95, 1033-1038.

Venti, C.A., Tataranni, P.A., & Salbe, A.D. (2005). Lack of Relationship between Calcium Intake and Body Size in an Obesity-Prone Population. *Journal of the American Dietetic Association*, 105, 1401-1407.

Welberg, J.W., Monkelbaan, J.F., De Vries, E.G., Muskiet, F.A., Cats, A., Oremus, E.T., Boersma-van, E.K., van Rijsbergen, H., van der Meer, R., Mulder, N.H., (1994). Effects of supplemental dietary calcium on quantitative and qualitative fecal fat excretion in man. *Annals of Nutritional Metabolism*, 38, 185–191.

White, K.M., Lyle, R.M., Flynn, M.G., Teegarden, D., & Donkin, S.S. (2006). The Acute Effects of Dairy Calcium Intake on Fat Metabolism During Exercise and Endurance Exercise Performance. *International Journal of Sport Nutrition & Exercise Metabolism*, 16, 565-579.

Xue, B., Greenberg, G., Kraemer, B., & Zemel, M.B. (2001). Mechanism of intracellular calcium ($[Ca^{2+}]i$) inhibition of lipolysis in human adipocytes. *The FASEB Journal*, 15, 2527-2529.

Xue, B., Moustaid-moussa, N., Wilkison, W.O., & Zemel, M.B. (1998). The agouti gene product inhibits lipolysis in human adipocytes via a Ca^{2+}-dependent mechanism. *The FASEB Journal*, 12, 1391-1396.

Zemel, M.B., Kim, J.H., Woychik, R.P., Michaud, E.J., Kadwell, S.H., Patel, I.R., & Wilkison, W.O. (1995). Agouti Regulation of Intracellular Calcium: Role in the Insulin Resistance of Viable Yellow Mice. *Proceedings of the National Academy of Sciences*, 92,, 4733-4737.

Zemel, M.B., Richards, J., Mathis, S., Milstead, A., Gebhardt, L., & Silva, E. (2005). Dairy augmentation of total and central fat loss in obese subjects. *International Journal of Obesity and Related Metabolic Disorders*, 29, 391-397.

Zemel, M.B., Shi, H., Greer, T., Dirienzo, G., & Paula C. (2000). Regulation of adiposity by dietary calcium. *The FASEB Journal*, 14, 1132-1138.

Zemel, M.B., & Sun, X. (2008). Calcitriol and energy metabolism. *Nutrition Reviews*, 66, S139-S146.

Zemel, M. (2003a). Calcium Modulation of Adiposity. *Obesity Research*, 11, 375-376.

Zemel, M.B. (1998). Nutritional and endocine modulation of intracellular calcium: Implications in obesity, insulin resistance and hypertension. *Molecular and Cellular Biochemistry*, 188, 129-136.

Zemel, M.B. (2001). Calcium Modulation of Hypertension and Obesity: Mechanisms and Implications. *Journal of the American College of Nutrition*, 20, 428S-4435.

Zemel, M.B. (2002). Regulation of Adiposity and Obesity Risk By Dietary Calcium: Mechanisms and Implications. *Journal of the American College of Nutrition*, 21, 146S-151.

Zemel, M.B. (2003b). Mechanisms of Dairy Modulation of Adiposity. *Journal of Nutrition*, 133, 252S-256.

Zemel, M.B. (2004). Role of calcium and dairy products in energy partitioning and weight management. *American Journal of Clinical Nutrition*, 79, 907S-9912.

In: Trends in Human Performance Research
Editors: M. Duncan and M. Lyons

ISBN: 978-1-61668-591-1
© 2010 Nova Science Publishers, Inc.

Chapter 10

ACTIVE VIDEO GAME PLAY – A NOVEL AND USEFUL EXERCISE MODALITY?

Mark Willems[*]
University of Chichester, UK

ABSTRACT

Exercise that meets guidelines for duration, frequency and intensity can provide health and performance benefits. Interactive video games or exergaming may thus provide an opportunity to enhance physical activity levels that would not normally be obtained with traditional means of exercise. This may be feasible taking into account the popularity of interactive games such as the Nintendo Wii Sports. In this chapter, studies will be reviewed that focussed on the physiological demands of Nintendo Wii Sports. Only studies that reported direct measurements of oxygen uptake or other means of predicting energy expenditure by playing Nintendo Wii Sports were discussed. Also, potential issues related to the physiological demands when playing Nintendo Wii Sports such as gender and body mass are identified. The main take home message from this chapter is that enhancement of human performance or

---

[*] Please address correspondence and requests for reprints to
Mark Willems,
Reader in Exercise Physiology, Faculty of Sport, Education & Social Sciences, University of Chichester, College Lane, Chichester, PO19 6PE, West Sussex, United Kingdom or e mail: m.willems@chi.ac.uk

improvement of health by regular interactive game play (i.e. exercise) must meet physiological requirements. It remains uncertain, however, whether individuals would intentionally implement regular interactive play to obtain health and performance benefits. Future work on physiological demands of playing interactive video games in the community may reveal the potential for enhancement of exercise performance and health.

Keywords: exercise, video game, energy expenditure, health.

INTRODUCTION

As of March 2009, Nintendo®, a video game company, sold 45.71 million copies of Wii Sports. It became the world's best-selling video game. More important, Nintendo Wii Sports is an interactive video game. It allows an individual to 'play' the sports boxing, tennis, baseball, golf or bowling. Considering the popularity of screen-based activities, interactive video game play or exergaming may provide an opportunity to enhance physical activity levels with screen activities (Daley, 2009; Maddison et al., 2007). Moreover, it offers an opportunity to enhance physical activity during recreational time in a home-based environment. As such, interactive video game play across the age span may provide individuals with levels of physical activity they would not otherwise acquire with traditional means of physical activity. Such potential impact has attracted the attention of exercise scientists and health promoters alike as there is convincing evidence that regular physical activity as part of an 'active' lifestyle can provide health benefits (Booth et al., 2008; Haskell et al., 2007). Why is this important? In light of the presence and rising incidence of obesity and type II diabetes in modern societies that is associated with at a substantial financial cost for health services, every opportunity for enhancing physical activity must be embraced to understand its potential impact, particularly considering the substantial evidence on the popularity of leisure screen time among children and adolescents. For example, leisure screen time in 80% of Canadian grades 6 to 10 exceeds the guidelines of 2 hrs (Mark et al., 2006). Many studies have also raised concern about the amount of entertainment time spend with 'screen-based inactivity' (Patriarca et al., 2009; Van den Bulck & Eggermont, 2006). According to a report by the Kaiser Family Foundation in 2004, "interactive games consume more than an hour daily of U.S. 8- to 18-year-olds' time". In the United Kingdom, the popularity is signified by the personal computer to be the most popular platform to play games across the age span (Pratchett, 2005). The report by Pratchett (2005) does not provide information on the time spend with interactive video game play. However, the popularity of interactive video game play in western societies is likely to increase rather than decline. Thus, regular play of interactive games may provide opportunities to influence weight management and risk factors for health. A potential additional impact of interactive video games is to become a training tool to enhance performance. However, in order for an interactive video game to have the potential to impact on performance or health, it is essential to quantify the physiological demands during game play.

Although a wide variety of interactive video games are available to the public in commercial and home-based environments, the aim of this chapter is to focus on acute physiological demands of Nintendo Wii Sports, primarily justified by its popularity as a household game. Peer-reviewed studies reporting the physiological demands of Nintendo Wii Sports were identified by searching Pubmed and SportDiscus in October 2009 (Table 1). Only studies were included that reported direct measurements of oxygen uptake or other means of predicting energy expenditure by playing Nintendo Wii Sports. This chapter will also attempt to consider potential issues related to the physiological demands when playing Nintendo Wii Sports. A key point of this chapter is that enhancement of human performance or improvement of health by regular interactive game play (i.e. exercise) must meet physiological requirements. It should be noted, however, that due to the demands of consumers linked with business interest of producers of active video games, some of the information in this chapter regarding Nintendo Wii Sports may have been already outdated as soon as new games enter the market. However, issues that will be identified that have an influence on the physiological demands when playing Nintendo Wii Sports may have general application for playing interactive video games.

NINTENDO WII SPORTS AND ENERGY EXPENDITURE

Nintendo Wii Sports is an interactive video game. Players use a wireless handheld movement sensing remote that is linked with an on-screen playable character. The movement of body parts and the movement sensing remote allow participation in the on-screen game. Therefore, due to the body movements, it is not surprising that the energy expenditure of playing Wii Sports uses significantly more energy than playing sedentary computer games

Table 1. Nintendo Wii Sports Studies

Study	Participants	Sample size	Games	Setting	Physiological outcome
Graves *et al.*, 2007	boys and girls (13-15 years)	6 boys, 5 girls	boxing, tennis, bowling	laboratory	predicted energy expenditure
Graves *et al.*, 2008	Boys and girls (11-17 years)	7 boys, 6 girls	boxing, tennis, bowling	laboratory	oxygen uptake, energy expenditure, heart rate
Barkley & Penko, 2009	adult males (35.7 ± 13.3 years) and females (27.3 ± 10.9 years)	6 males, 6 females	boxing	laboratory	oxygen uptake, heart rate,
Graf *et al.*, 2009	boys and girls (10-13 years)	14 boys, 9 girls	boxing, bowling	laboratory	oxygen uptake, heart rate, expired ventilatory rate
Lanningham-Foster *et al.*, 2009	children (9-15 years) and adults (18-56 years)	11 boys, 11 girls, 10 males, 10 females	boxing	laboratory	oxygen uptake
Willems & Bond, 2009	young-adults (21.0 ± 1.0 years)	7 males, 3 females	boxing, baseball and tennis	laboratory	oxygen uptake, heart rate

(Barkley & Penko, 2009; Graves *et al.*, 2007; Lanningham-Foster *et al.*, 2009), rest (Graf *et al.*, 2009; Lanningham-Foster *et al.*, 2009), or rest while watching television (Lanningham-Foster *et al.*, 2009, Graf *et al.*, 2009). In the study by Graves *et al.* (2007), it was reported that the predicted energy expenditure was at least 51% higher in boys and girls, aged 13-15 years, during active gaming of either boxing, tennis or bowling compared to sedentary gaming. This was the first study reporting the physiological demands of Nintendo Wii Sports. Energy expenditure was predicted by an IDEEA (i.e. intelligent device for energy expenditure and activity) system, a system acknowledged by the authors not detecting arm movements well (Graves *et al.*, 2007). However, in another study by the same group, a portable indirect calorimetry system (i.e. MetaMax 3B) was used for measurement of oxygen uptake (Graves *et al.*, 2008). In that study, bowling, tennis and boxing were played for 15 minutes each with 5 minutes seated rest between games. Tennis and boxing are externally paced games involving screen opponents whereas bowling is a self-paced game. Boxing had the highest energy expenditure compared with tennis and bowling. The values for oxygen uptake in Graves *et al.* (2008) were 0.55 ± 0.17 $L \cdot min^{-1}$ for Wii bowling, 0.61 ± 0.19 $L \cdot min^{-1}$ for Wii tennis and $0.82 \pm .40$ $L \cdot min^{-1}$ for Wii boxing. Clearly, boxing provided the highest energy expenditure but the data also showed that boxing had the largest variation. Such variation may complicate general conclusions about the usefulness of particular interactive video games. Interestingly, the energy expenditure of the games bowling, boxing and tennis was best predicted with hip activity, measured by accelerometry, and least by heart rate. Heart rate information is commonly used by exercisers to monitor intensity but this parameter may not be useful for establishing intensity of interactive game play. The differences between the Wii Sports tennis and bowling was primarily due to play requirements allowing more limb activity when playing tennis (Graves *et al.*, 2008). In addition, the increased energy expenditure of boxing compared with tennis and bowling was due to the game requirement of boxing to use both arms (Graves *et al.*, 2008). Wii boxing in the study by Graf *et al.* (2009) also led to higher energy expenditure for boys (2.9 fold) and girls (3.3 fold), aged 10-13 years, than rest. It was further observed that the step rates of boxing and bowling were low confirming that it was primarily upper body movements that accounted for energy expenditure (Graf *et al.*, 2009). Thus, there is still potential to enhance energy expenditure of Wii boxing by providing clear instructions on lower body movements. Interestingly, the energy expenditure for boxing was similar between boys and girls but higher in boys for bowling (Graf *et al.*, 2009). An influence of gender on the energy expenditure was also highlighted by Barkley and Penko (2009) but was absent for Wii boxing, tennis and bowling in Graves *et al* (2008) study. In the study by Barkley and Penko (2009) a comparison of energy expenditure of 6 adults males and 6 adult females showed higher energy expenditure for boxing in males. It was argued that potential differences in aggressive behaviour may have resulted in more vigorous arm movements of males (Barkley & Penko, 2009). Potential individual and gender differences in energy expenditure by interactive game play may complicate drawing general conclusions. In addition, differences in gender and body mass highlight that individual variation in energy expenditure during boxing, for example, may influence the potential of these games to impact performance or health. Future studies may want to examine the differences between energy expenditure as a function of body mass in children as energy expenditure is associated with body mass during weight-bearing activities. Thus, playing Nintendo Wii Sports raises energy expenditure above rest. Because the energy expenditure of some traditional activities is known to be sufficient to provide health benefits, a comparison of Nintendo Wii Sports with traditional activities would allow a better understanding and interpretation of the potential impact of regular game play on health.

NINTENDO WII SPORTS VS TREADMILL WALKING

Studies have compared the energy expenditure of Nintendo Wii Sports with treadmill walking (Barkley & Penko 2009, Graf *et al.,* 2009, Willems & Bond, 2009). Graf *et al* (2009) assessed the energy expenditure of Nintendo Wii bowling (15 min) and boxing (15 min) and compared this with treadmill walking at 2.6, 4.2 and 5.7 km/h in 23 healthy children (14 boys, 9 girls) aged 10-13 years. Wii boxing had energy expenditure similar or greater than walking at 4.2 and 5.7 km/h. Nintendo Wii bowling also resulted in higher oxygen uptake values in boys due to a higher footstep rate. There was no difference in footstep rate between boys and girls when playing Nintendo Wii boxing, this potentially explaining the similarity in energy expenditure between boys and girls for boxing. More important, the study by Graf *et al* (2009) showed that treadmill walking, an activity for which energy expenditure is primarily caused by lower body movements, could result in equal energy expenditure to interactive video game play by primarily upper body movements such as boxing. This observation may have implications for clinical populations with a limitation for lower body movement. It would allow such individuals to achieve energy expenditure with upper body movements when playing interactive games that are commonly achieved with whole body exercise.

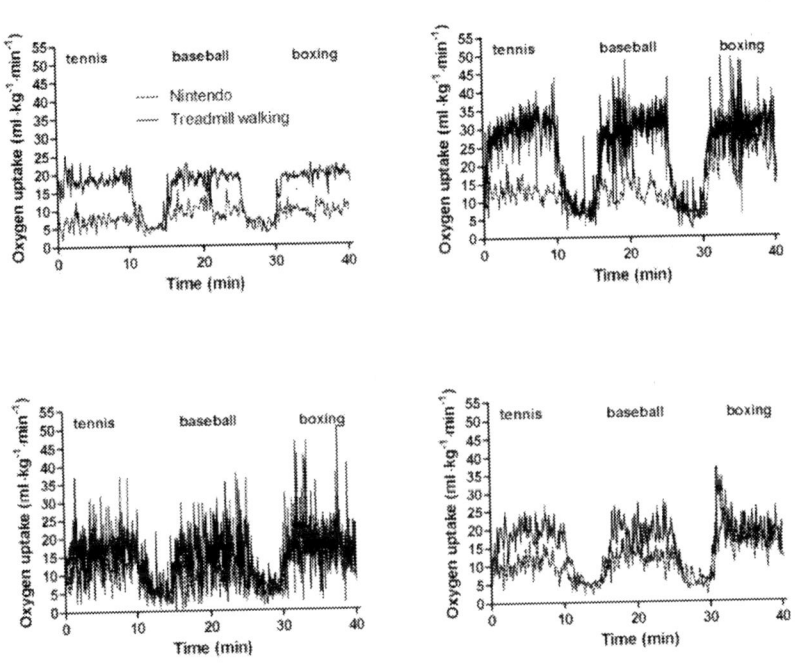

Figure 1. Oxygen uptake as a function of time for four participants during 3 bouts of 10 minutes of brisk treadmill walking and 3 bouts of 10 minutes play on Nintendo Wii Sports tennis, baseball and boxing.

Figure 1 shows the oxygen uptake traces of four male subjects as recorded by the portable metabolic system Cosmed K4b^2. The Cosmed K4b^2 is a breath-by-breath sampling method recording the oxygen values in ml·min^{-1}. The traces were normalized for each individual's body weight (i.e. ml·kg^{-1}·min^{-1}). The individuals played the Nintendo Wii Sports tennis, baseball and boxing each for 10 min or walked for similar time periods on a treadmill at a self-selected fast walking speed (see Willems & Bond, 2009). To ensure ecological validity, the participants received instructions to play Wii Sports at their own game level or to walk fast on the treadmill. Substantial individual variation can be observed for the oxygen traces. Some have matching oxygen uptake for the Wii Sports (tennis, baseball and boxing) and self-paced fast treadmill walking

(Figure 1C). Another subject was consistently having higher values during walking (Figure 1A). The overall result from that study was that the oxygen uptake (and therefore energy expenditure) of boxing was not significantly different than self-paced fast treadmill walking (Willems & Bond, 2009). Movements of upper and lower body were not recorded in that study and these factors may have explained the individual responses to interactive game play. However, the variation may also reveal that a recommendation for the health benefits of particular Wii Sports based on known physiological data may not be as straightforward as it seems.

NINTENDO WII SPORTS: IMPLICATIONS FOR PERFORMANCE?

A consideration for the potential implication of interactive video games for training or health effects needs to take into account the physiological demands of the exercise. It is essential for the exercise (or interactive video game) to meet the principles for exercise training to improve performance (Wenger & Bell, 1986). The effects of exercise training on aerobic fitness, for example, result from the interplay of intensity, frequency and duration of the exercise bouts. Age needs to be considered as the American College of Sports Medicine recommends for adults a heart rate of 60% of maximum to improve and maintain aerobic fitness whereas for young people, the intensity must be higher than 80% of heart rate (Baquet et al., 2003). As yet, no studies have examined the potential of interactive video games in replacement for conventional training methods. Interestingly, a study by Warburton et al (2007) with adult males (average BMI making them overweight) found improvements in maximum oxygen uptake related to frequency of combined cycling exercise on a Gamebike® while playing a choice of Sony Playstation 2® video games. This study was not based on principles of training as the intensity and duration were not controlled. However, adherence was higher resulting in increased time being physically active. Addiction of children and adolescents to video games exists (Chiu et al., 2004). However, the extent to which addiction to active video game play may have a positive effect on adherence is not known. It is of interest to understand causal factors for 'beneficial' addiction which can be used to stimulate active video game play in children and adolescents who do not normally participate in traditional means of physical activity. Motivation why people play interactive video games needs further examination (Chin A Paw *et al.*, 2008; Epstein *et al.*, 2007). Health psychologists should improve our understanding on adherence issues of active video game play. At this point, it would be extremely speculative whether interactive video games should be promoted as exercise training tools. Adherence issues and boredom with playing games in addition to the absence of obeying principles of training with playing interactive video games may limit the potential of interactive video games to be a training tool to achieve cardiovascular improvements and enhance performance. However, manufacturers could be encouraged to build in feedback that allow individuals to control the intensity level of interactive game play as is common for traditional exercise devices such cycle ergometers and treadmills in public fitness facilities. Such facilities may then justify providing exergaming fitness.

NINTENDO WII SPORTS: IMPLICATIONS FOR HEALTH?

In 2007, Haskell *et al* published the consensus statement of the American Heart Association and the American College of Sports Medicine on physical activity and health. In the consensus statement, the use of the metabolic equivalent as an indicator for exercise intensity was advocated as it allows a calculation of the accumulated MET·min·wk^{-1} for combinations of moderate (3-6 METs) and vigorous intensity (6 METs and higher) exercise. One metabolic equivalent (MET) is defined as the energy cost of a 70 kg, 40 year old man at rest (Byrne *et al.*, 2005). However, as pointed out by Byrne *et al* (2005), substantial variation exists between individuals with respect to their resting energy cost. A measurement of an individual's resting energy expenditure was suggested to measure accurately the energy cost during activity. It was recognized by Haskell *et al* (2007) that actual MET values during exercise may vary from person to person but may work for the purpose of recommendation for the general population. It was recommended that individuals should aim to accumulate an energy expenditure of 450 to 750 MET·min·wk^{-1}. Several studies on Nintendo Wii Sports have quantified the MET values in health individuals. The metabolic cost of Wii boxing for adults was 4.4 ± 1.3 METs (Barkley & Penko, 2009), 4.7 ± 1.4 METs for young adults (Willems & Bond, 2009) and 3.2 ± 1.4 METs for adolescents (Graves *et al.*, 2008). Although the average MET value for boxing in all studies was between 3-6 METs, categorizing boxing as a moderate-intensity exercise, the variation in the study by Graves *et al* (2008) indicated not all individuals met the required intensity. Participants in Graves et al (2008) study were six girls and seven boys aged 11-17. In contrast, boxing by young-adults who were not receiving instructions regarding body movements, indicated that the MET value of only 1 participant was below 3.0 (Willems & Bond, 2009). Other Wii Sports provided lower METs values (Graves *et al.*, 2007; Willems & Bond, 2009). Therefore, Nintendo Wii boxing when played regularly seems to have the potential to provide health benefits at least in young-adults. It would be interesting to examine the metabolic cost of interactive video game play in special (e.g. 'sedentary' elderly) and clinical populations. In those populations, the required intensity of the exercise may be lower in order to achieve health benefits. In addition, some may argue that a lack of appropriate levels of physical activity may be regarded as a pre-clinical condition for the onset of chronic diseases. Interestingly, Murphy *et al* (2009) examined the effects of interactive game play on risk factors for chronic diseases in overweight children with endothelial dysfunction and reported improved endothelial function. Endothelial dysfunction is an early event of atherogenesis (Gimbrone *et al.*, 2000) with known beneficial effects by traditional exercise programmes in healthy males (Clarkson *et al.*, 1999) and in overweight children and adolescents (Kelly *et al.*, 2004).

IN SUMMARY

Although particular interactive video game play has potential for performance and health benefits, it is uncertain whether individuals would intentionally implement regular play to obtain those benefits. Adherence of active video game play in social-recreational environments is also not known making the impact of active video games on community health mere speculation. However, future studies are warranted to examine the potential benefits of interactive game play in clinical populations (e.g. cancer) as the requirements for exercise to obtain health benefits may be less than what is required for those that are considered healthy. Individuals with mobility impairments of the lower body may benefit from playing 'intense' interactive video games with upper body movements. Evidence in support on positive long-term effect of active video game play is emerging but most studies to date have dealt with the acute physiological effects of active video game play. Considering the popularity of interactive video games, it is anticipated that future work on physiological demands of playing interactive video games in the community may reveal the potential for enhancement of exercise performance and health.

REFERENCES

Baquet, G., van Praagh, E. & Berthoin, S. (2003). Endurance training and aerobic fitness in young people. *Sports Med*, 33, 1127-1143.

Barkley, J. E. & Penko, A. (2009). Physiologic Responses, Perceived Exertion, and Hedonics of Playing a Physical Interactive Video Game Relative to a Sedentary Alternative and Treadmill Walking in Adults. *JEPonline*, 12, 12-22.

Booth, F. W., Laye, M. J., Lees, S. J., Rector, R. S. & Thyfault, J. P. (2008). Reduced physical activity and risk of chronic disease: the biology behind the consequences. *Eur J Appl Physiol*, 102, 381-390.

Byrne, N. M., Hills, A. P., Hunter, G. R., Weinsier, R. L. & Schutz, Y. (2005). Metabolic equivalent: one size does not fit all. *J Appl Physiol*, 99, 1112-1119.

Chiu, S. I., Lee, J. Z. & Huang, D. H. (2004). Video game addiction in children and teenagers in Taiwan. *Cyberpsychol Behav*, 7, 571-581.

Chin A Paw, M. J., Jacobs, W. M., Vaessen, E. P., Titze, S. & van Mechelen, W. (2008). The motivation of children to play an active video game. *J Sci Med Sport*, 11, 163-166.

Clarkson, P., Montgomery, H. E., Mullen, M. J., Donald, A. E., Powe, A. J., Bull, T., Jubb, M., World, M. & Deanfield, J. E. (1999). Exercise training enhances endothelial function in young men. *J Am Coll Cardiol*, 33, 1379-1385.

Daley, A. J. (2009). Can exergaming contribute to improving physical activity levels and health outcomes in children? *Pediatrics*, 124, 763-771.

Gimbrone, M. A. Jr, Topper, J. N., Nagel, T., Anderson, K. R. & Garcia-Cardeña, G. (2000). Endothelial dysfunction, hemodynamic forces, and atherogenesis. *Ann N Y Acad Sci*, 902, 230-239.

Graf, D. L., Pratt, L. V., Hester, C. N. & Short, K. R. (2009). Playing active video games increases energy expenditure in children. *Pediatrics*, 124, 534-540.

Graves, L., Stratton, G., Ridgers, N. D. & Cable, N. T. (2007). Comparison of energy expenditure in adolescents when playing new generation and sedentary computer games: cross sectional study. *BMJ*, 335, 1282-1284.

Graves, L. E., Ridgers, N. D. & Stratton, G. (2008). The contribution of upper limb and total body movement to adolescents' energy expenditure whilst playing Nintendo Wii. *Eur J Appl Physiol*, 104, 617-623.

Haskell, W. L., Lee, I. M., Pate, R. R., Powell, K. E., Blair, S. N., Franklin, B. A., Macera, C. A., Heath, G. W., Thompson, P. D. & Bauman, A. (2007).

Physical activity and public health: updated recommendation for adults from the American College of Sports Medicine and the American Heart Association. *Circulation*, 116, 1081-1093.

Kelly, A. S., Wetzsteon, R. J., Kaiser, D. R., Steinberger, J., Bank, A. J. & Dengel, D. R. (2004). Inflammation, insulin, and endothelial function in overweight children and adolescents: the role of exercise. *J Pediatr*, 145, 731-736.

Maddison, R., Mhurchu, C. N., Jull, A., Jiang, Y., Prapavessis, H. & Rodgers, A. (2007). Energy expended playing video console games: an opportunity to increase children's physical activity? *Pediatr Exerc Sci*, 19, 334-343.

Mark, A. E., Boyce, W. F. & Janssen, I. (2006). Television viewing, computer use and total screen time in Canadian youth. *Paediatr Child Health*, 11, 595-599.

Murphy, E. C., Carson, L., Neal, W., Baylis, C., Donley, D. & Yeater, R. (In Press). Effects of an exercise intervention using Dance Dance Revolution on endothelial function and other risk factors in overweight children. *Int J Pediatr Obes*.

Patriarca, A., Di Giuseppe, G., Albano, L., Marinelli, P. & Angelillo, I. F. (2009). Use of television, videogames, and computer among children and adolescents in Italy. *BMC Public Health*, 9, 139.

Pratchett, R., Harris, D., Taylor, A. & Woolard, A. (2005). *Gamers in the UK: Digital Play, Digital Lifestyles*. London: BBC.

Van den Bulck, J. & Eggermont, S. (2006). Media use as a reason for meal skipping and fast eating in secondary school children. *J Hum Nutr Diet*, 19, 91-100.

Wenger, H. A. & Bell, G. J. (1986). The interactions of intensity, frequency and duration of exercise training in altering cardiorespiratory fitness. *Sports Med*, 3, 346-356.

Willems, M. E. T. & Bond, T. S. (2009). Metabolic equivalent of brisk walking and playing new generation active computer games in young-adults. *Med Sport*, 13, 95-98.

In: Trends in Human Performance Research
Editors: M. Duncan and M. Lyons

ISBN: 978-1-61668-591-1
© 2010 Nova Science Publishers, Inc.

Chapter 11

AUGMENTED ECCENTRIC LOADING: THEORETICAL AND PRACTICAL APPLICATIONS

Philip H. Watkins[*]
University of Derby, UK

ABSTRACT

The purpose of this paper is to examine the efficacy of using augmented eccentric loading (AEL) as an alternative training approach for athletes and weight trainers involved in strength and power development. The practice of incorporating AEL into resistance exercise is still relatively new and although limited, there is evidence that supports the contention that AEL may lead to both superior acute and chronic adaptations over more traditional methods. AEL involves coupled concentric and overloaded eccentric muscle actions, and attempts to optimise the muscular adaptations associated with stretch-shortening cycle (SSC) activities. Examples of exercises that can be performed with an eccentric-enhanced resistance include: plyometric drop/depth jumps,

---

[*] Please address correspondence and requests for reprints to
Philip H. Watkins,
School of Science, University of Derby,
Kedleston Road, Derby, United Kingdom, DE22 1GB
E mail p.h.watkins@derby.ac.uk

jumps in place, squats, squat jumps, lunges, bench press and bench throws. Due to the 'stop-start' nature of AEL exercises, cluster set configurations (i.e., inter-repetition rest intervals) maybe used as a means for implementing AEL into a periodised training plan. The inter-repetition rest interval may improve the quality of each AEL repetition when compared with more traditional set structures by offsetting the affects of fatigue. More research into concentric and eccentric *relative* loading as well as the *rate* of eccentric loading is necessary to further define its role within the weight training and strength and conditioning communities. However, it is possible that enhanced training effects may be achieved if increased eccentric loads are implemented into periodised strength-training programs.

Keywords: Augmented Eccentric Loading (AEL), Stretch-Shortening Cycle (SSC), Plyometrics, Muscle Spindle, Golgi Tendon Organ (GTO), Muscle Tendon Unit (MTU), Cluster Sets.

INTRODUCTION

Human movement is made possible through the relative contributions of eccentric, isometric and concentric muscle actions (Moore et al., 2007). The muscular forces produced during maximal eccentric actions are greater than during maximal concentric or isometric actions (Enoka, 1996; Hortobagyi et al., 1996). This combination of muscle actions is termed a stretch-shortening cycle (SSC), where performance maybe enhanced by a prior countermovement (Doan et al., 2002). Elasticity of muscles and tendons has also shown to improve performance in SSC movements (Wilson & Flanagan, 2008; Wilson et al., 1994), its importance in sprinting and jumping (Kryolainen & Komi, 1995) characterised by a fast eccentric muscular stretch, followed immediately by a powerful, concentric muscular contraction. Using a stretch immediately prior to a concentric action increases the concentric phase, resulting in increased force production, power output (van Ingen Schenau et al., 1997; Komi & Bosco, 1978) and shift in the force-velocity curve to the right (Komi, 1986). The majority of strength and power programs however, focus on developing concentric one-repetition maximum (1-RM) force production, and often overlook the benefits of using increased eccentric loads (Doan et al., 2002) on the musculature. Additionally, 40% to 50% greater force can be produced during the eccentric phase compared with the concentric phase of exercise (Dudley et al., 1991), indicating that the eccentric muscle action is *underloaded* during traditional isoinertial weight training (Yarrow et al., 2008). An alternative form of strength training, termed augmented eccentric loading (AEL) involves coupled concentric and overloaded eccentric muscle actions, and attempts to optimise the muscular adaptations associated with resistance exercise (Kaminski et al, 1998). This paper aims to examine the efficacy of using AEL as an alternative training approach and provides a practical example for its implementation into a periodised strength-training program.

A Brief Overview of the Literature

Augmented Eccentric Loading (AEL) has been defined as 'the application of a heavy eccentric force immediately prior to a relatively lighter concentric force' (Moore et al., 2007). The benefits of such additional eccentric loads being most prevalent during the early stages of the concentric phase (Newton et al, 1997) of an SSC movement. Augmented eccentric forces may be provided either by i) increasing the rate of muscle lengthening or ii) by increasing the relative load or a combination of the two.

Influencing the Rate of Eccentric Loading

Early AEL studies (Cronin et al., 2001; Bobbert et al., 1996) found that performing depth jumps from incrementally higher displacements were more effective at acutely increasing vertical jump height when compared with countermovement jumps (Bobbert et al., 1996). These findings are subject to an athlete's ability to absorb force upon landing, since the AEL during depth jumping increases accelerative force, impulse (i.e., the product of force (F) and the change in time (Δt) during the application of that force), and the rate of muscle lengthening upon landing (Moore et al., 2007). Toumi et al (2004) reported similar findings following a study into the effects of eccentric phase velocity of plyometric training on vertical jump performance. Participants performed tests for maximal isometric and concentric squat force as well as squat and countermovement jump displacement, before and after an 8 week experimental speed squat training protocol, with eccentric speeds of 0.2 m/s and 0.4 m/s. Both groups' squatting and jumping performances improved significantly following the intervention, however, a reduction in the amortisation rate of the speed squat was also reported in the 0.4 m/s group.

The superior adaptations of the group using the faster eccentric action was attributed to the increased eccentric loading via the rapid stretch imposed on the muscle. Conversely, Moore et al (2007) investigated the acute effects of AEL on jump squat performance. Thirteen resistance-trained men (age = 22.8 ± 2.9 years) were assessed performing jump squats under 4 experimental conditions (condition 1, 30% 1-RM back squat; conditions 2, 3 and 4, jump squats with a 30% 1-RM subsequent to the application of AEL conditions of 20, 50 and 80% of 1-RM back squat respectively). Results indicated that peak velocity, force and power values obtained during the jump squats were similar ($p > 0.05$) across all loading conditions. However, the eccentric portion of the jump squat in this study was executed at a relatively slow velocity (Moore et al., 2007), serving to reduce any additional accelerative force. Therefore, the *rate* of eccentric action may be more significant than absolute load, possibly explaining why the loading parameters were ineffective in this study.

Increasing the Relative Eccentric Load

Doan et al (2002) measured the acute effects of AEL on subsequent concentric 1- repetition maximum (RM) strength in the bench press exercise. Eight moderately trained men (mean age, 23.9 yrs) performed maximal attempts in the bench press using detaching hooks (i.e., weight releasers) which allowed them to lower 105% of their concentric 1-RM and raise 100%. All participants significantly ($p = 0.008$) increased their 1-RMs by 5 to 15 pounds with the mean bench press score increasing from 97.44kg for the normal eccentric condition to 100.57kg for the AEL condition. Although limited by a lack of sensitive measures, such as force, power and rate of force development (RFD), the results demonstrated that additional eccentric loading maybe beneficial in producing acute increases in 1-RM bench press. The loadings used in this study were of particular interest, maximal concentric barbell loads were coupled with a small AEL of 105% of concentric 1-RM, whereas the concentric barbell loadings used by Moore et al (2007) were significantly smaller (30% 1-RM), with AEL ranging from 20 to 80% 1-RM. The authors of this study (Moore et al., 2007) suggested the possibility of the existence of a concentric load threshold, below which, AEL may be ineffective at improving performance. More research using multiple concentric loads is required to determine if such a threshold exists.

Brandenburg & Docherty (2002) compared the effects of 2 strength training programs on maximal strength of the elbow flexors in 23 resistance trained males over a 9 week period. Participants' were randomly assigned to either a dynamic constant external resistance (DCER) (performing 4 sets of 10 repetitions at 75% of concentric 1-RM) or a dynamic accentuated external resistance (DAER) (performing 3 sets of 10 repetitions at 75% of concentric 1-RM with eccentric actions performed at a load of approximately 110-120% of concentric 1-RM) group. Resistances were adjusted to match concentric and eccentric strength. Participants' in both groups trained 2 times per week for the first 2 weeks and then 3 times per week for the remainder of the 9 week training period. Both groups reported improvements in elbow flexor strength and elbow extensor strength ($p<0.05$), however, the DAER group produced significantly greater development in elbow extensor strength compared with DCER training. The authors attributed these differences within the DAER group to the pennate muscle fibre design of the elbow extensors (i.e., conducive to high force production) compared with the parallel fibre design of the elbow flexors.

Yarrow et al (2008) evaluated neuroendocrine responses and strength adaptations to 5 weeks of traditional (TRAD) and eccentric-enhanced (AEL) progressive resistance training. Twenty-two previously untrained men (22 ± 0.8 years) completed 1 familiarisation and 2 baseline bouts, 15 exercise bouts (i.e., 3 times per week for 5 weeks) and 2 post-intervention testing bouts. Participants were randomly assigned into TRAD (4 sets of 6 repetitions at 52.5% 1-RM) or AEL (3 sets of 6 repetitions at 40% 1-RM concentric and 100% 1-RM eccentric) groups. Both groups experienced similar increases in bench press (~ 10%) and squat (~ 22%) strength during the intervention. At the conclusion of training, post-exercise total testosterone (TT) and bioavailable testosterone (BT) concentrations increased (~ 13% and 21 % respectively, $p<0.05$) and growth hormone (GH) concentrations increased (~ 750-1200%, $p < 0.05$) acutely following exercise in both protocols. Post-exercise lactate accumulation was similar between both groups. However, blood lactate concentrations for the AEL group were significantly lower 30 to 60 minutes into recovery. This study concluded that TRAD and AEL training appeared to result in similar muscular strength adaptations and neuroendocrine responses, whilst post-exercise lactate clearance was enhanced following AEL training. The findings are inconsistent with a variety of studies that have reported increases in strength following 1 to 9 weeks of AEL training (Friedman et al., 2004; Brandenburg & Docherty, 2002; Hortobagyi et al., 2001). However, this study suggests that AEL maybe a suitable alternative to TRAD training and may have population-specific benefits.

SUMMARY

There is evidence to support the hypothesis that AEL may produce superior strength gains (i.e., both acute and chronic) over more traditional methods in both untrained and resistance trained populations. Much of the conflict within the literature however, is possibly due to methodological differences, for example, inconsistencies in training volumes and intensities, modes of assessment and subject populations. It appears that superior strength gains have been achieved when eccentric loads have been in excess of the concentric 1-RM (i.e., ~105-120% of the concentric 1-RM) or when faster eccentric actions attribute (i.e., rate dependent interactions) to an augmentation in eccentric loading via the rapid stretch imposed on the muscle. More research into the role of concentric and eccentric loading as well as the rate of eccentric loading is necessary in particular, concentric load thresholds across populations. Manipulations to AEL protocols may also yield favourable training adaptations with increases in training volume and duration across the training cycle. Athletes and strength trainers with limited time to participate in resistance exercise may also benefit from AEL, as similar improvements in muscular strength have occurred at lower training volumes and time commitment when compared with more traditional methods. Additionally, AEL may benefit specific muscle groups over others, and may aid recovery in some populations.

PHYSIOLOGICAL MECHANISMS

The mechanisms underlying muscular adaptations following AEL have not been fully determined (Yarrow et al., 2008). Kraemer & Ratamess (2005) have suggested that post-exercise alterations in testosterone or growth hormone influence skeletal muscle hypertrophy, although the degree to which these anabolic hormones influence augmentations in muscle hypertrophy remains unknown. Four physiological mechanisms have been theorised as being potential contributors to enhanced concentric performance following AEL (Cronin et al, 2001; Bobbert et al, 1996).

1. Increased Neural Stimulation:

During AEL, when muscles are forcibly stretched, their tension rises sharply, resulting in more motor units being recruited (Moore et al., 2007). Quick and forceful eccentric actions cause increases in the excitability of proprioceptors for an optimal reaction by the neuromuscular system, resulting in a more forceful concentric action. These changes are controlled and partially counterbalanced by two proprioceptors that are most relevant in SSC movements, muscle spindles and golgi tendon organs (GTOs) (Watkins, 2009). Located in the intrafusal fibres and innervated by gamma-motor neurons, muscle spindles are facilitatory mechanoreceptors that react to changes in muscle length to protect the muscle-tendon complex (Flanagan & Comyns, 2008). The inevitable unloading of the muscle spindle during muscle shortening is counteracted by a concomitant shortening of the intrafusal muscle fibres. This stretch reflex occurs during the yielding phase (when the hip, knee and ankle joints are flexing), and compensates for muscle exposed to forcible stretches (Watkins, 2009). Located in the extrafusal fibres and innervated by alpha motor neurons (Rieman & Lephart, 2002), GTOs act as a protective mechanism, responding to changes in tension rather than length, inhibiting agonist muscles and facilitating the antagonist muscles (Brooks et al., 2000). When muscle contractile forces reach a point where damage to the muscle-tendon complex may occur, GTOs increase afferent activity through inhibition of the motor neurons that innervate the stretched muscles, whilst simultaneously exciting the motor neurons of the antagonist muscles (Rieman & Lephart, 2002; Brooks et al., 2000). Plyometric training (e.g., AEL) can upregulate the stretch reflex, as well as reduce the inhibitory reflexes (Watkins, 2009; Jensen et al., 1991).

2. Stretching of the Parallel and Series Musculotendinous Complex:

A second mechanism suggests that elastic energy stored in the series elastic elements (SEEs) in the eccentric phase is re-used during the concentric phase (Watkins, 2009). An increased rate of eccentric loading may result in a brief storage of additional elastic energy, which may then be used during the concentric phase. At the onset of shortening, elastic recoil of these elements add to the work output of the muscle-tendon complexes involved in these actions (Walshe et al., 1998). Tendon recoil speeds are much greater than muscle shortening speeds, exercises with increasing stretching loads result in a reduction in muscle activation and surface EMG (Ebben et al., 2008; Schmitdbleicher, 1992) indicating an increased reliance on the elastic properties of the musculotendinous unit (MTU) during ballistic actions.

3. The Elastic Nature of Tendons:

Muscle force production increases during the eccentric phase of SSC movements, resulting in the time available for force development being greater (Zatsiorsky & Kraemer, 2006) than in concentric only movements. There is very little lengthening of the muscles in this eccentric phase, and at the moment of transition (reversibility) from lengthening to shortening, the force is developed under isometric conditions, so the influence of high velocity is avoided (Wilson & Flanagan, 2008). A continuation of tendon lengthening enables a body to continue to drop downward (Zatsiorsky & Kraemer, 2006). The control of the MTU stiffness has been shown to play an important role in making full use of the benefits of SSC movements (Kubo et al., 1999). When no external forces are present these systems maintain a constant shape, however when acted upon by external forces they generate elastic force to oppose the external force and store and return elastic energy (Latash & Zatsiorsky, 1993). A stiffer spring-like action in the legs allows humans to run with higher stride frequencies than otherwise possible (Ferris & Farley, 1997). Tendon stiffness is constant, however, the stiffness of muscle is variable and depends upon the forces exerted. Such tendons work as springs, and allow for storing and recoiling large amounts of mechanical energy at each step (Zatsiorsky & Kraemer, 2006). Harrison et al (2004) demonstrated that sprinters used a stiffer leg spring at any given speed when compared with high calibre endurance athletes but suggested that endurance athletes may benefit from the inclusion of SSC related activities in their training. Superior athletes can develop high forces, and the stiffness of their muscles when active exceeds the stiffness of their tendons. It has been proposed that the influence of the facilitatory reflex which originates from the muscle spindles can be enhanced through training and can improve muscle stiffness (Watkins, 2009). The role of the inhibitory force feedback component (from the GTOs) can be simultaneously decreased (Komi, 1992). It appears that MTU stiffness is an important variable for superior performance in SSC movements (Wilson et al, 1994).

4. Preloading:

The significance of developing pre-tension before muscle shortening has been reported in the literature (Hortobagyi et al., 2001; Helgeson & Gajdosik, 1993). AEL may allow a portion of the cross-bridges to be attached prior to concentric action, thereby increasing joint moments early in the concentric phase (Bobbert et al., 1996). Concentric movements that are immediately preceded by either isometric or eccentric actions lead to greater concentric torque when compared with purely concentric actions (Walshe et al., 1998; Jensen et al., 1991).

According to the force-velocity relationship, force must be developed when velocity is slow in order to achieve very high forces. Higher levels of muscle activation earlier in the movement allow muscles to produce greater forces over a range of joint angles thereby optimising performance (Butler et al., 2005; Bobbert et al., 1996). In most high speed movements, muscle force is developed in isometric conditions (Zatsiorsky & Kraemer, 2006) through much of the movement, with the magnitude of lengthening and shortening of muscles depending upon the amplitude of the eccentric and concentric phases and the muscle involved. This near isometric contraction of the muscles allows large forces to be generated in accordance with the force-velocity relationship, as well as operate near their optimal length.

IMPLEMENTING AEL INTO A PERIODISED TRAINING PLAN

AEL training requires the athlete to perform coupled concentric and overloaded eccentric muscle actions (Yarrow et al., 2008) and efficacy for using AEL in athlete training appears promising (Yarrow et al., 2008; Brandenburg & Docherty, 2002; Doan et al., 2002; Hortobagyi et al., 1996). It may be necessary for athletes to include a practice phase (e.g., 1-3 sessions) to ensure optimal familiarisation and jumping proficiency. This may assist in overcoming technical flaws and less-than-optimal volition due to the AEL. Examples of AEL exercises include: plyometric drop/depth jumps (one- and two-legged), jumps in place, squats, squat jumps, lunges, bench press and bench throws. Due to the 'stop-start' nature that is inevitable when performing AEL exercises (resulting from the inter-repetition 'set-up' of bands, dumbbells, weight releasers etc), cluster set configurations maybe used as a means for implementing AEL into a periodised training plan (see Table 1).

Table 1. Example cluster set structure for the back squat (i.e. with a load-related AEL) during a basic strength phase of a periodised training plan

Type of Cluster	Exercise	Sets x Repetitions	Cluster set repetition loading structure (i.e., % eccentric/concentric 1-RM/repetition)	Inter-repetition rest interval (s)
Standard	Back Squat with AEL (e.g., using weight releasers)	4-6 x 6/1 4-6 x 6/2 4-6 x 6/3	105/80/1 105/80/1 105/80/1 105/80/1 105/80/1 105/80/1 105/80/2 105/80/2 105/80/2 105/80/3 105/80/3	30 30 30

Notes: 6/1 = 6 total repetitions broken down into 6 clusters of 1; 6/2 = 6 repetitions broken down into 3 clusters of 2; 6/3 = 6 total repetitions broken into 2 clusters of 3. In the above example, each set has an average eccentric intensity of 105% of concentric 1-RM and a concentric intensity of 80% of 1-RM for the back squat. These can be periodised over the phase of training. Inter-repetition rest intervals can be shortened or lengthened up to 45 seconds depending upon the training goals and the athlete's level of development.

Traditionally, a training set is comprised of a series of repetitions performed in a continuous fashion. A cluster set however, may employ a 15-45 second rest period between each repetition, the main manipulation involving modifications to the inter-repetition rest interval (e.g., 10/1 = 10 total repetitions in the set with inter-repetition with the selected inter-repetition rest between each repetition or 10/2 = 10 total repetitions in the set with the selected inter-repetition rest after each series of 2 repetitions) (Table 2). Other modifications may include variations to individual loading patterns contained in the set or alternating the number of repetitions employed. The inclusion of inter-repetition rest intervals could improve the quality of individual repetitions when compared with traditional set structures, and offset the affects of fatigue on performance by enabling the athlete to partially recover between each repetition (Haff et al., 2008a). Manipulations to the cluster repetition scheme, inter-repetition rest interval length and the loading sequence should be matched to the phase of training, training goals, and the performance characteristics of the sport (Haff et al., 2008b). Exercise selection and progression must be guided by training status, untrained participants have been reported to respond to the eccentric phase of a high stretch load with a period of inhibition (Sale, 1992).

Table 2. Example cluster set structure for plyometric drop jumps (i.e., with a velocity related AEL) during a basic power phase of a periodised training plan

Type of Cluster	Exercise	Sets x Repetitions	Cluster set repetition loading structure (i.e., Box height/repetition)	Inter-repetition rest interval (s)
Standard	Plyometric Drop Jump with AEL (e.g., using viper belt with bands)	1-3 x 10/1 1-3 x 10/2 1-3 x 10/3	40/1 40/1 40/1 40/1 40/1 40/1 40/1 40/1 40/1 40/1 40/2 40/2 40/2 40/2 40/2 40/5 40/5	5 10 15

Notes: 10/1 = 10 total repetitions broken down into 10 clusters of 1; 10/2 = 10 repetitions broken down into 5 clusters of 2; 10/5 = 10 total repetitions broken into 2 clusters of 5. During the eccentric phase, intensity can be altered by changing the height of the box (e.g., 40cm in the above example), or increasing/decreasing the number of bands attached to the belt. The bands are released immediately prior to the concentric phase of the jump. Rest intervals can be lengthened up to 45 seconds depending upon the training goals and the athlete's level of development.

Velocity-related AEL activities such as drop jumps use rapid powerful movements that are preceded by a pre-loading countermovement. Coaches should encourage rapid, powerful movements that reduce the eccentric/concentric transition times from their athletes as well as emphasise the importance of minimising ground contact times.

CONCLUSION

The principle of specificity determines the demands required in any sport or physical activity, combining exercises that demand variation in movement velocities, coupled concentric and overloaded eccentric muscle actions (AEL), and targeting different phases of the SSC, may provide superior performance results. Similarly, efficient use of elastic energy is probably the key mechanism behind increases in movement speed, power and efficiency observed in SSC movements. Examples of exercises that can be adapted to provide an augmented eccentric load include: plyometric drop/depth jumps (one- and two-legged), jumps in place, squats, squat jumps, lunges, bench press and bench throws. The inter-repetition rest interval may improve the quality of each AEL repetition when compared with more traditional set structures by offsetting the affects of fatigue. More research into concentric and eccentric *relative* loading as well as the *rate* of eccentric loading is necessary to further confirm its role within the weight training and strength and conditioning communities. AEL maybe a suitable alternative to TRAD training and may have population-specific benefits. It is possible that enhanced training effects could be achieved if increased eccentric loads are implemented into periodised strength-training programs. Consideration should be given to exercise selection, variation, training intensity and volumes throughout the program as well as the training status of the athlete.

REFERENCES

Bobbert, M, Gerritsen., K. Litjens, M. & van Soest A. J. (1996). Why is the countermovement jump height greater than squat jump height? *Medicine and Science in Sports and Exercise*, 28, 1402-1412.

Brandenburg, J.P., & Docherty, D. (2002). The effects of accentuated eccentric loading on strength, muscle hypertrophy and neural adaptations in trained individuals. *Journal of Strength and Conditioning Research*, 16, 25-32.

Brooks, G. A., Fahey, T., White, T. & Baldwin, K. M. (2000). *Exercise Physiology: Human Bioenergetics and its Applications.* Mountain View, CA: Mayfield Publishing.

Butler, R.J., Crowell, H. & Davis, I. (2003). Lower extremity stiffness: Implications for performance and injury. *Clinical Biomechanics*, 18, 511-517.

Cronin, J.B., McNair, P. & Marshall, R. (2001). Magnitude and decay of stretch-induced enhancement of power output. *European Journal of Applied Physiology*, 84, 575-581.

Doan, B.K., Newton, R., Marsit, J., Triplett-McBride, N., Koziris, L., Fry, A. & Kraemer, W. (2002). Effects of increased eccentric loading on bench press 1-RM. *Journal of Strength and Conditioning Research*, 16, 9-13.

Dudley, G.A., Tesch, P., Miller, B. & Buchannan, P. (1991). Importance of eccentric actions in performance adaptations to resistance training. *Aviation Space Environmental Medicine*, 62, 543-550.

Ebben, W.P., Simenz, C. & Jensen, R. (2008). Evaluation of plyometric intensity using electromyography. *Journal of Strength and Conditioning Research*, 22, 3, 861-868.

Enoka, R.M. (1996). Eccentric contractions require unique activation strategies by the nervous system. *Journal of Applied Physiology*, 81, 2339-2346.

Ferris, D.P. & C.T. Farley (1997). Interaction of leg stiffness and surface stiffness during human hopping. *Journal of Applied Physiology*, 82, 15-22.

Flanagan, E.P. & Comyns, T.M. (2008). The use of contact time and the reactive strength index to optimize fast stretch-shortening cycle training. *Strength and Conditioning Journal*, 30, 32-38.

Friedman, B., Kinscherf, R., Vorwald, S., Muller, H., Kucera, H., Borisch, S., Richter, G., Barsch, P. & Billeter, R. (2004). Muscular adaptations to computer guided strength training with eccentric overload. *Acta Physiologica Scandinavia*, 182, 77-88.

Haff, G., Burgess, S. & Stone, M. (2008a). Cluster training: theoretical and practical applications for the strength and conditioning professional. *Professional Strength and Conditioning Journal*, 12, 12-16.

Haff, G. Whitley, A., McCoy, L. B., O'Bryant, H., Kilgore, J., Haff, E., Pierce, K. & Stone, M. (2008b). Cluster training: a novel method for introducing training program variation. *Strength and Conditioning Journal*, 30, 67-76.

Harrison, A.J., Keane, S. & Coglan, J. (2004). Force-velocity relationship and stretch shortening cycle function in sprint and endurance athletes. *Journal of Strength and Conditioning Research*, 18, 473-479.

Helgeson, K. & Gajdosik, R. (1993). The stretch-shortening cycle of the quadriceps femoris muscle group measured by isokinetic dynamometry. *Journal of Orthopaedics and Sports Physical Therapy*, 17, 17-23.

Hortobagyi, T., Devita, P. Money, J. & Barrier, J. (2001). Effects of standard and eccentric overload strength training in young women. *Medicine and Science in Sports and Exercise*, 33, 1206-1212.

Jensen, R.C., Warren, B., Lauresen, C. & Morrissey, M. (1991). Static pre-load effect on knee extensor isokinetic concentric and eccentric performance. *Medicine and Science in Sports and Exercise*, 23, 10-14.

Kaminski, T.W., Wabberson, C. & Murphy, R. (1998). Concentric versus enhanced eccentric hamstring strength training: clinical implications. *Journal of Athletic Training*, 33, 216-221.

Komi, P.V. (1992). Stretch-Shortening Cycle. In: *Strength and Power in Sport*. P.V. Komi, ed. Blackwell Science.

Komi, P.V. (1986). The stretch-shortening cycle and human power output. In: *Human Muscle Power*. N.L. Jones, N. McCartney and A.J. McComas, eds. Champaign, IL: Human Kinetics.

Komi, P.V. & Bosco, C. (1978). Utilization of stored elastic energy in leg extensor muscles in men and women. *Medicine and Science in Sport and Exercise*, 10, 261-265.

Kraemer, W.J. & Ratamess, N.A. (2005). Hormonal responses and adaptations to resistance exercise and training. *Sports Medicine*, 35, 339-361.

Kryolainen, H. & Komi, P. (1995). The neuro-muscular system in maximal stretch-shortening cycle exercises: Comparison between power and endurance trained athletes. *Journal of Electromyography and Kinesiology*, 5, 15-25.

Kubo, K., Kawakami, Y. & Fukunaga, T. (1999). Influence of elastic properties of tendon structures on jump performance in humans. *Journal of Applied Physiology*, 87, 2090-2096.

Latash, M.L. & Zatsiorski, V. (1993). Joint stiffness: myth or reality? *Human Movement Science*, 12, 653-692.

Moore, C.A., Weiss, L.W., Schilling, B.K., Fry, A.C. & Li, Y. (2007). Acute effects of augmented eccentric loading on jump squat performance. *Journal of Strength and Conditioning Research*, 21, 372-377.

Newton, R.U., Murphy, A.J., Humphries, B.J., Wilson, G.J., Kraemer, W.J. & Hakkinen, K. (1997). influence of load and stretch shortening cycle on the kinematics, kinetics and muscle activation during explosive upper body movements. *European Journal of Applied Physiology and Occupational Physiology*, 75, 333-342.

Riemann, B. & Lephart, S. (2002). The sensorimotor system, part 1: the physiologic basis of functional joint stability. *Journal of Athletic Training*, 37, 71-79.

Sale, D.G., (1992). Neural Adaptations to Strength Training. In: *Strength and Power in Sport*. P.V. Komi (ed). Blackwell Science.

Schmitbleicher, D. (1992). Training for Power Events, In: *The Encyclopedia of Sports Medicine, Vol 3: Strength and Power in Sport*. P.V.Komi, ed. Oxford, UK: Blackwell

Toumi, H., Best, T.M., Martin, A., Guyer, S.F. & Poumart, G. (2004). Effects of eccentric phase velocity of plyometric training on the vertical jump. *International Journal of Sports Medicine*, 23, 391-398.

Van Ingen Schenau, G.J., Bobbert, M. & De Haan, A. (1997). Does elastic energy enhance work and efficiency in the stretch shortening cycle? *Journal of Applied Biomechanics*, 13, 389-415.

Walshe, A.D., Wilson, G. & Ettema, G. (1998). Stretch-shorten cycle compared with isometric pre-load: contributions to enhanced muscular performance. *Journal of Applied Physiology*, 84, 97-106.

Watkins, P.H. (2009). *The Stretch Shortening Cycle: A Brief Overview*. In: M.J. Duncan and M. Lyons (eds) Advances in Strength and Conditioning Research. New York: Nova Science Publishers.

Wilson, J.M. & Flanagan, E. (2008). The role of elastic energy in activities with high force and power requirements: A brief review. *Journal of Strength and Conditioning Research*, 22, 1705-1715.

Wilson, G.J., Murphy, A., & Pryor, J. (1994). Musculotendinous stiffness: its relationship to eccentric, isometric and concentric performance. *Journal of Applied Physiology*, 76, 2714-2719.

Yarrow, J.F., Borsa, P., Borst, S., Sitren, H., Stevens, B. & White, L. (2008). Early-phase neuroendocrine responses and strength adaptations following eccentric-enhanced resistance training, *Journal of Strength and Conditioning Research*, 22, 1205-1214.

Zatsiorsky, V.M. & Kraemer, W. (2006). *Science and Practice of Strength Training*. Human Kinetics (2nd Edition).

In: Trends in Human Performance Research
Editors: M. Duncan and M. Lyons

ISBN: 978-1-61668-591-1
© 2010 Nova Science Publishers, Inc.

Chapter 12

PREDICTORS OF EXERCISE PERFORMANCE

*Ahmad Alkhatib**
University Campus Suffolk, UK

ABSTRACT

The prediction of exercise performance depends on the type of performance and the metabolic energy provided from aerobic and anaerobic energy sources. Exercise intensity affects both respiratory and metabolic physiological parameters. Therefore, selected physiological measurements at maximal and submaximal exercise intensity provide accurate tools for exercise testing and training. Maximal oxygen uptake reflects the maximum aerobic capacity and is accepted as the best single measure for exercise performance. Respiratory measures at submaximal intensities determine the transition between moderate and heavy intensity domains and indentify anaerobic threshold. Lactate response to exercise intensity helps to identify intensities at lactate threshold, which is useful to predict performance. Those intensities correspond to maximal lactate steady state in constant load tests. However, wide range intensities at lactate threshold and several identified thresholds make their use in prescribing exercise challenging. Recent metabolic concepts involved

---

* Please address correspondence and requests for reprints to
Ahmad Alkhatib,
School of Health, Science and Social Care,
University Campus Suffolk, Neptune Quay, Ipswich, IP4 1QJ
E mail a.alkhatib@ucs.ac.uk

identifying the cross-over point between relative fat and carbohydrate utilisation, and the intensity at maximal fat oxidation. Interrelationships combining metabolic and respiratory measurements may provide an integrative role to predict exercise performance, and understand the underlying factors regulating and limiting metabolism and performance. A recently proposed model has described relative carbohydrate utilisation as a function of blood lactate concentration. The model adds to the understanding of integrated metabolic factors that limit exercise performance, and may be a useful predictor, though further research is needed.

Keywords: Exercise intensity, Blood lactate concentration, relative rates of carbohydrate and fat utilisation.

AN OVERVIEW ON EXERCISE PERFORMANCE

Human exercise tolerance can be predicted by physiological parameters which are dependant on the type of exercise performance and metabolic energy provided from aerobic or anaerobic resources. The limitations to provide metabolic energy aerobically and anaerobically depends on generating ATP as the metabolic energy source. Depending on the energy system, maximal and submaximal physiological testing have evolved, and relevant concepts in exercise testing and prescription predicted exercise performance. For example, the adaptations to endurance exercise have been shown to enhance the ability to perform maximal and submaximal exercise and the ability to achieve peak power in endurance type events (Howley et al. 1995). Therefore, measurements for maximal and submaximal exercise performance have been developed to provide accurate tools for exercise testing and prescription. This chapter will focus on reviewing the latest research trends in exercise performance predictors especially endurance performance, and how each predictor can be used to for exercise testing and training.

Maximal aerobic energy is reflected by the measurements of maximal oxygen uptake (VO_{2max}) which represents the functional limits to the cardiovascular and respiratory systems. VO_{2max} reflects training status, and achieving VO_{2max} reflects high levels of lactic acid in the blood, elevated respiratory exchange ratio (RER), and age estimated maximal heart rate (Howley et al., 1995). Blood lactate concentration (BLC) is one of the most often measured parameters during performance testing of athletes and during clinical exercise testing (Goodwin et al., 2007). Reflecting both aerobic and anaerobic performance, BLC response is probably the most accurate measure of exercise performance and its levels have been indicative of both submaximal and maximal exercise levels (Brooks, 1985). Thus, different lactate thresholds have been determined using a single incremental exercise test (Wasserman *et al.* 1973), and more recently BLC response has been characterised at different exercise intensities on separate occasions using the concept of maximal lactate steady state (MLSS), (Beneke, & vonDuvillard, 1996).

The generation of ATP is also dependant on the metabolic substrates of fat and carbohydrate, and exercise intensity determines the relative utilisation rates. Thus, the interaction between fat and carbohydrate utilisation during exercise has been studied extensively, and metabolic concepts based on the relative rates between fat and carbohydrates (CHO) have evolved as a tool to describe the adaptations to endurance training (Brooks and Mercier, 1994). Recently introduced concepts included the cross-over point (COP), which represents the power output at which energy derived from CHO predominates over that of fatty acids (Brooks and Mercier, 1994). The exercise intensity at which fat oxidation is maximal (Fatmax) has also been introduced recently and shown to be a useful predictor for submaximal exercise intensities (Achten *et al.*, 2002; Venables *et al.*, 2005).

Biochemical interrelationships between those exercise performance predictors has been attempted to better understand them and facilitate exercise testing (Bircker *et al.*, 2005, Jeukendrup *et al.*, 2004). An interrelationship between lactate, carbohydrate and fatty acid during exercise has been developed (Alkhatib, & Beneke, 2008a, Beneke *et al.*, 2009), and shown to serve as an independent explanatory factor for the inter-individual variability in fat and CHO metabolism (Alkhatib and Beneke, 2008b, Alkhatib & Beneke, 2008c), and independently of pedalling rate and age (Beneke *et al.* 2009, Alkhatib *et al.*, 2005). However, the practical applications of the latter concepts in exercise testing and prescription and in training require further research.

HOW EXERCISE INTENSITY AFFECTS SELECTED PHYSIOLOGICAL MEASUREMENTS OF PERFORMANCE

Exercise intensity refers to how hard the body is working during physical activity. Exercise intensity is mostly represented as the external power output measured in watts (W). This becomes meaningful when considering the corresponding oxygen uptake response which includes the internal work or the resting metabolic rate. Exercise intensity is commonly used in relative terms to VO_{2max} as (%VO_{2max}), or to peak power output (%). Both terms are commonly used interchangeably, with it important to state that % VO_{2max} is higher than % peak power as it includes resting metabolic rate in its percentage. The following review examines the physiological responses of oxygen uptake (VO_2), carbon dioxide production (VCO_2), blood lactate, and the substrate utilisation of CHO and fat to exercise at both local muscle, and whole body levels.

EFFECTS OF EXERCISE INTENSITY ON OXYGEN UPTAKE AND CARBON DIOXIDE OUTPUT

Exercise intensity determines different respiratory responses of VO_2 consumption and a corresponding VCO_2 production. The oxygen cost of performing work depends on the work rate. In an incremental exercise test VO_2 essentially increases linearly as exercise intensity increases. Jones and Pool (2005) reported a VO_2 slope of 10 $ml.min^{-1}.W^{-1}$ in a 3-min stage incremental test for trained subjects. This linear relationship of VO_2-power output was not affected by altering the incremental test protocol in terms of the increment size and workload or subjects' fitness level (Beaver et al., 1986; Howley et al., 1995; Wasserman et al., 2005; Jones, & Poole, 2005).

In constant work load tests three temporal components characterise the VO_2 response and are reportedly divided into moderate, heavy and severe intensity domains (Gaesser, & Poole, 1996). Some investigators have divided the VO_2 responses into four by adding the very heavy exercise intensity domain (Ozyener et al., 2001). Furthermore, the time course of the change in VO_2 response within each intensity domain has also been characterised and attributed to a different stimuli. Three temporal components characterises the VO_2 response: a) the early, usually rapid response; b) the slower, exponential increase; and c) the steady state (Whipp, 1994). In healthy subjects, it takes approximately 30s to attain 63%, 60s to attain 86%, and 120s to attain 98% of the steady state amplitude of VO_2 (Jones, & Poole 2005). A steady state attainment of VO_2 of > 99%, is reached by approximately 3 min at moderate exercise intensity. At higher intensities in the heavy and severe domains, VO_2 continues to increase beyond the 4th min, and so, the rate at which VO_2 increases is greater the higher the work rate, and an influence of a slow component is expected in the heavy, and severe intensity domains (Jones, & Poole, 2005). VO_2 continues to increase in the severe exercise intensity until the point of fatigue, and the maximum level of VO_2 or VO_{2max} is attained at the end of exercise (Xu and Rhodes, 1999).

VCO_2 during exercise comes from three sources: a) aerobic metabolism, which is linearly related to VO_2; b) bicarbonate buffering of lactic acid; and c) acute hyperventilation as respiratory compensation of pulmonary capillary blood (Stringer et al., 1995). Therefore, VCO_2 response is similar to that of VO_2 below lactate threshold (LT) but increases disproportionately at higher intensities above LT. VO_2 was mostly described using two regression lines as in the commonly used V-slope method for the estimation of anaerobic threshold (Beaver et al., 1986), though some investigators do not support the existence of a threshold (Yeh et al., 1983), and some described VCO_2 as an exponential function of exercise intensity (Dennis and Noakes, 1992).

VCO_2 is considered to reach a steady state after approximately 3 min depending on exercise intensity (Stringer et al., 1995). It has been argued that VCO_2 has a slower response than that of the VCO_2 at moderate and heavy exercise intensity domains. This is reflected by a lower delay time and a lower time constant for VCO_2 compared with that of VCO_2 as shown in Bell et al. (1999), and explained in details in Whipp & Ward (1993) and in Whipp (2006).

Increased exercise intensity elicits increases in VO_2 and VCO_2, reflecting the following mechanisms (Wasserman et al., 2005):

1) Increase in VO_2 needed to satisfy the increased work of respiratory muscles and the heart at high ventilatory and cardiac output responses.
2) Increased recruitment of fast-twitch muscle fibres.
3) Increased muscle recruitment in terms of muscle groups and number.
4) Acidemia facilitating O_2 unloading from haemoglobin by shifting the oxyhaemoglobin dissociation curve downward for a given PO_2.
5) Progressive vasodilatation to the local muscle units by metabolic vasodilators (e.g. high H^+ gradient, High PCO_2, low PO_2), thereby, increasing O_2 flow and consumption at O_2 deficient sites.
6) The O_2 cost of converting lactate to glycogen in the liver, as the lactate concentration rises, is also contributory.

LACTATE RESPONSE TO EXERCISE INTENSITY

At physiological pH, lactic acid almost completely dissociates to hydrogen and lactate ions, therefore the terms lactic acid and lactate are often used synonymously. However, when describing lactate-lactic acid transport across membranes precise terminology is required (Brooks, 1985). Blood lactate concentration (BLC) is dependant on work load essentially, but highly related to exercise duration, fitness level, age, and cardiovascular disease status (Wasserman *et al.*, 2005). Attempts to describe lactate response to exercise focused mainly on the intensity at which BLC threshold is achieved, and many mathematical models have been introduced for this purpose (Beaver *et al.*, 1986; Wasserman *et al.*, 1990). A progressive incremental load testing in which the workload is increased every 1-4 min until exhaustion is the most common method to detect lactate response for performance and clinical exercise testing (Goodwin *et al.*, 2007).

Lactate response remains similar to its resting levels or increases slightly at low exercise intensities. However, BLC starts to increase abruptly at any intensity between about 40-80% VO_{2peak}. The main two approaches describing BLC response to exercise can be classified as the bilinear model (Beaver *et al.*, 1986) and the mono-exponential model introduced by Hughson *et al.* (1987). Wasserman *et al.* (1990) argued that the bilinear model fits the BLC data better than the exponential at intensities corresponding to BLC values below 4 $mmol.l^{-1}$. This is mainly because of better distribution of the parameters' extremes being estimated at lower exercise intensities. However, 3-parameter mono-exponential model has been preferred when describing BLC over the whole range of exercise intensities in incremental tests (Dennis *et al.*, 1992, Alkhatib, & Beneke, 2005). The level of increment size and duration have a clear effect on BLC attainment of a steady state (Stockhausen *et al.*, 1997). Therefore, some investigators suggested performing constant load tests lasting longer than 20 min at several exercise intensities, to determine the time course of BLC (Beneke and von Duvillard, 1996, Beneke, 2003, Billat *et al.*, 2003).

MECHANISMS OF LACTATE INCREASE AND ACCUMULATION

The understanding of the lactate role has changed significantly during the past 30 years. Gladden (2000) summarised that the shift in the knowledge moved from lactate being known as an immediate energy donor for muscle contraction; a primary factor in muscle soreness; the central cause of O_2 debt; and a causative agent in muscle fatigue into the following:

1. Cell Redox

Traditionally it was argued that muscle and blood lactate concentrations increase with exercise intensity because of inadequate O_2 supply to the exercising muscles (muscle hypoxia) since the era of Hill *et al.* (1924). This belief was developed later that century by Margaria *et al.* (1933), whom suggested that lactate increase during exercise was related to the O_2 debt. This theory is currently being considered and strongly supported by several experiments (Wasserman *et al.*, 1985; Wasserman *et al.*, 1973). The latter group of investigators related the concept of anaerobic threshold to cell redox. Their concept states that at certain intensity lactate increases in the cell because of the mitochondrial proton shuttle. This normally oxidises cytosolic $NADH + H^+$ as it transfers protons and electrons to mitochondrial O_2, and is too slow to reoxidise the reduced cytosol NAD. This process results in the faster conversion of pyruvate to lactate leading to lactate accumulation.

2. Mass Action

When glycolysis proceeds at a faster rate than pyruvate can be utilised by the mitochondrial tricarboxylic acid cycle. This results in elevated pyruvate levels in the cytosol, and consequently lactate accumulation by mass action (Spriet *et al.*, 2000). Contributing factors to mass action include an increased catecholamine hormones which increase glycolytic rate, and also the increased recruitment of fast twitch glycolytic motor units (Xu and Rhodes, 1999).

3. Imbalance between Lactate Production and Removal

Brooks *et al.* (2005) demonstrated that the majority of lactate formed by muscle contraction is not converted to glycogen in the skeletal muscle but oxidised by a variety of tissues including skeletal muscle, heart muscle, and possibly other organs such as the brain tissues. Rather than causing oxygen debt, Brooks *et al.* (2005) suggest this process actually pays it off.

LACTATE AS A PREDICTOR OF EXERCISE PERFORMANCE

Lactate response to exercise is arguably the most accurate predictor of exercise endurance performance and BLC has become a standard measure for exercise intensity since the turn of the 20th century (Hill *et al.*, 1924). LT is the most often measured parameter in exercise testing for athletes and also clinical testing (Goodwin *et al.*, 2007). LT is determined by performing an incremental load test and collecting several blood samples every (commonly 3) minutes until volitional exhaustion. Thus the workload corresponding to LT is identified. However, several points can be identified that vary from approximately 1.0 to 8.0 $mmol.l^{-1}$ (Stegmann, & Kindermann, 1981), and several methods have been proposed to identify an individual threshold or a fixed lactate point and several reviews have thoroughly discussed the specific methods of identification LT (Goodwin *et al.*, 2007).

Prolonged constant load tests are able to detect the highest BLC can be reached over time and the highest corresponding workload. The highest blood lactate concentration that can be maintained over time in a constant-load test without continual blood lactate accumulation is termed maximal lactate steady state (MLSS) (Beneke, & vonDuvillard, 1996), and the corresponding workload is termed MLSS workload or intensity. Training at MLSS-workload (velocity) has been shown to improve performance indicators of VO_{2peak}, velocity at VO_{2peak}, time to exhaustion, and MLSS-velocity, and this was coupled with no change in MLSS, which was approximately 4 $mmol.l^{-1}$ (Billat *et al.*, 2004).

Billat (2004) suggested that at MLSS-intensity correspond to approximately 90% of relative CHO utilisation, and a respiratory quotient of around 0.95 - 1.0. MLSS varies between individuals from 2 - 8 $mmol.l^{-1}$ (Billat *et al.*, 2003; Beneke *et al.*, 2000), and reflects variations in exercise intensities of approximately 55 - 85% VO_{2peak} (Beneke, 2000, Billat *et al.*, 2004). Therefore, investigating the metabolic changes that modulate MLSS and MLSS-intensity, merits further research.

EFFECTS OF EXERCISE INTENSITY ON THE UTILISATION OF FAT AND CARBOHYDRATE

Fat and CHO are the principle substrates that fuel human skeletal muscles at rest and during exercise. The energy from fat and CHO is used for muscle contraction for ATP regeneration. Although protein is a viable source of energy, it is not used to fuel the energy needs of the body at any appreciable extent, except during starvation. The contribution of the oxidation of some amino acids, such as branched chain amino acids and leucine, contribute to sustaining endurance exercise, and may be increased by training (Brooks, 1987 in Brooks, & Mercier, 1994). However, the overall energy flux rates change little, suggesting that fat and CHO are the predominant fuels during exercise (Henderson *et al.*, 1985; Brooks, 1987; Rennie *et al.*, 1994; in Brooks, & Mercier 1994).

It is well documented that the relative utilisation of fat and CHO can vary enormously and depends on many factors such as dietary and nutritional status (Bergman, & Brooks 1999), exercise mode (Kang *et al.*, 2004), intensity and duration (Romijn *et al.*, 1993), training status (Coyle *et al.*, 1997) and hormonal milieu (Winder *et al,.* 1979 in Ranallo, & Rhodes, 1998). However, exercise intensity appears to be the main factor that relates to all of the latter effects (Achten *et al.*, 2002).

Exercise intensity affects storage and the relative use of fat and CHO. Fat utilisation during exercise tends to be highest at low exercise intensities, and declines gradually coupled with a gradual increase in CHO utilisation as exercise intensity increases. Exercise intensities between 30-65 % VO_{2peak} tend to elicit the highest fat utilisation, and higher intensities of approximately 85 % VO_{2peak} tend to elicit minimal fat oxidation, and almost total dependence on CHO utilisation (Spriet, 2002, Romijn *et al.*, 1993, Brooks & Mercier 1994, Achten *et al.*, 2002, Gonzalez-Haro *et al.*, 2007).

Romijn *et al.* (1993) demonstrated that plasma Free Fatty Acids (FFAs) turnover accounts for the fats metabolised during low exercise intensities between 25 - 40 % VO_{2max}. However, muscle triglycerides contribution increases as the contribution of plasma FFAs slightly decreases at intensity of 65 % VO_{2max}. At higher exercise intensities such as 85 % VO_{2peak} total fat oxidation decreases as well as plasma FFA sources allowing increases in energy sources of CHO (glycogen and glucose).

Thus, FFAs utilisation depends on essentially on exercise intensity. Plasma FFAs are able to supply most substrate at low intensities, but a limited substrate source at higher intensities. It has not yet been established why the use of FFAs is restricted at those exercise intensities. However, below is a summary of the most viable explanations.

THE POSSIBLE MECHANISMS OF THE DECLINE IN FAT METABOLISM IN FAVOUR OF CARBOHYDRATE METABOLISM

A) Fat Regulates Carbohydrate Metabolism

It has been proposed that the reduction in muscle carbohydrate oxidation rate was caused by high plasma FFA in resting muscles (Randle *et al.*, 1963 in van Loon *et al.*, 2001). The latter concept related the increased availability of plasma FFAs to suppressing pyruvate dehydrogenase complex (PDH) activation, via rise in mitochondrial acetyle-CoA/CoA ratio, and by decreasing glycolytic flux, via the inhibitory effects of high citrate concentrations on phosphofructokinase activity. Therefore, this concept suggests that the relative utilisation of fat and CHO is determined by the availability of plasma FFAs. However, later studies did not find any connection between FFA availability and the reduction in fat oxidation at high intensity exercise (Romijn *et al.*, 1993, van Loon *et al.*, 2001).

B) Carbohydrate Regulates Fat Metabolism

It has been shown in isolated, contracted and perfused muscles that high CHO availability is associated with reduced long chain fatty acid (LCFA) oxidation (Hargreaves, & Spriet, 2006). The latter researchers reported several studies in rodent and human muscles suggesting that high CHO availability decreases LCFA oxidation (Dyke *et al.*, 2001, Sidossis *et al.*, 1997, Turcotte *et al.*, 2002, in Hargreaves, & Spriet, 2006), though this was not observed elsewhere (Yee *et al.*, 2001 in Hargreaves, & Spriet, 2006). In contrast, low CHO availability impair muscle oxidative metabolism because the shift to oxidise fat as the predominant fuel either reduces the production rate of acetyl-CoA or results in an inability to maintain an adequate level of Krebs cycle intermediates. Thus, CHO availability plays an important role in regulating fat oxidation.

Some suggested that increased glycolytic flux rate can directly inhibit FFAs oxidation by either phosphorylating it by its AMP activated kinase (Winder, 2001), or by glucose inhibitory effects on LCFA (Coyle *et al.*, 1997). It has been suggested that the cellular mechanism for the decrease in LCFA oxidation at rest is linked to an increase in the glycolytic flux and to a subsequent increase in levels of malonyl-CoA (Ruderman *et al.*, 1999, Turcotte *et al.*, 2002 in Hargreaves, & Spriet, 2006). High levels of malonyl-CoA inhibit carnitine palmitoyltrasferase-I (CPT-I) activity in the cytosol which limits the FFA entry into the mitochondria, and reduces LCFA oxidation (McGarry *et al.*, 1983). Therefore, it has been suggested that high glycolytic flux rates during high intensity exercise indirectly limit LCFA causing down-regulation of CPT-I (Saggerson, 1981, in Starritt *et al.*, 2000, Van Loon *et al.*, 2001).

There are several factors that can determine the level of CPT-1, among which Acetyl-CoA/ CoA (Constantin-Teodosiu, *et al.*, 1998), reduction in pH (Starritt, *et al.*, 2000), or the decline in the free carnitine due to increased acetylation (increased acetyle-carnitine) (van Loon, *et al.*, 2001). Starritt, *et al.* (2000) explained that the accumulations of acetyl-CoA, free co-enzyme A, and acetylcarnitine do not counteract the malonyl-CoA induced inhibition of CPT-I activity, and small decreases in pH produce large reductions in the activity of CPT-I and may contribute to the decrease in fat metabolism that occurs during moderate and intense aerobic exercise intensities. Thus, the current knowledge in this area seem to suggest that the inhibition of CPT-1 is due to either decline in free carnitine pool, or a decrease in intracellular pH (van Loon, *et al.*, 2001).

Increased exercise intensity increases catecholamine hormones causing higher glycolytic flux, and increased CHO oxidation (Brooks, & Mercier, 1994). The increase in the glycolytic flux is also associated by lactate accumulation. It has been shown that lactate, pyruvate, or both, can directly inhibit lipolysis (Boyd, *et al.*, 1974).

An increased availability of pyruvate increases has been suggested to be an important trigger for PDH activation among others such as Ca^{+2} concentration, NAHAD/NAD, ATP/ADP, and acetyl-CoA-Co ratios, leading to increased CHO oxidation (Spriet, & Heigenhauser, 2002). On the other hand, a reduction in pyruvate availability has been associated with reduced CHO oxidation (Mourtazakis *et al.*, 2006). Thus, it may be considered that CHO availability can directly or indirectly determine the rate of fat oxidation and regulate the fuel interaction during exercise.

FAT AND CARBOHYDRATE AS PREDICTORS OF PERFORMANCE

Understanding of the mechanisms of fat and CHO interaction during different exercise intensities is very important for health and exercise performance. It has been shown that fuel selection abnormality is associated with metabolic diseases like type-2 diabetes, and obesity (Kelly, & Simoneau, 1994, Martin *et al.*, 1995, Colberg *et al.*, 1995, in van Loon, *et al.*, 2001). Furthermore, it has been suggested that a reduced capacity to oxidise fat is an important factor in developing obesity and type-2 diabetes. This was investigated in Pima Indians who showed higher rate of weight gain due to an elevated 24-h RQ (Zurlo *et al.*, 1990 in Jeukendrup, & Wallis 2005). The latter subjects have been reported more prone to obesity and type-2 diabetes associated with reduced capacity to oxidise fat, and insulin resistance, because of a change in their lifestyle into a more Western lifestyle (Kelly & Goodpaster, 2001 in Jeukendrup & Wallis, 2005). Reduced FFA utilisation in obese subjects and subjects with a risk of obesity has been characterised by: a) decrease in lipoprotein lipase; b) decrease in CPT-I and in citrate synthase, which leads to a reduced FFAs transfer into the mitochondria. Exercise training induces metabolic changes that are favourable for the diagnosis, prevention, and treatment of obesity, and therefore was recommended for clinicians and health practitioners (The House of Common Health Committee, 2004).

Exercise training is known to induce metabolic changes that improve substrate selection. It has been established that an increased capacity of trained muscles to oxidise blood-borne FFAs and TGs, along with an increased capacity to access intramuscular TGs, results in glycogen sparing and increased exercise endurance capacity (Mole *et al.*, 1971 Henriksson & Reitman 1977, Oscai *et al.*, 1982, Hollozy, & Coyle, 1984, Gollnick, 1985; in Brooks, & Mercier, 1994). Muscle glycogen sparing is known to be a limiting factor in endurance performance especially in heavy exercise intensities and events lasting 1 hour or longer (Below *at el.*, 1995, Hargreaves, 2004). Glycogen availability and sparing are known to be favourable factors to prolong exercise performance, and glycogen depletion has been implicated in fatigue (Below *et al.*, 1995, Hargreaves, 2004). The latter summarised that muscle glycogen is an important fuel for contracting skeletal muscle during prolonged strenuous exercise, and its availability has several roles among which are the resynthesis, excitation-contraction coupling, insulin action and gene transcription may be all dependent on glycogen availability during exercise. On the other hand, low muscle glycogen is linked with reduced muscle glycogenolysis; increased glucose and non-esterified FFA uptake and protein degradation; accelerated glycogen resynthesis; impaired excitation-contraction coupling; enhanced insulin action and potentiation of the exercise-induced increases in transcription of metabolic genes (Hargreaves, 2004). Recent research has suggested that carbohydrate sensing via mouth rinsing reduces fatigue rate through an activation of brain regions, especially the anterior cingulated cortex and striatum (Chambers *et al.*, 2009).

Theoretical concepts that are based on the interaction between fat and carbohydrate metabolism have developed rapidly during the last 15 years. Brooks and Mercier (1994) reviewed CHO and fat interaction with exercise intensity as they defined the cross over concept as the power output at which energy derived from CHO sources predominates over energy from lipids (Figure 1). On the other hand, the exercise intensity that elicit maximal fat oxidation has recently been defined (Achten *et al.*, 2002, Venables *et al.*, 2005). Since then, "metabolic" training at the cross-point has been suggested to improve performance, and that the ability to improve the power output at the cross-point may improve performance (Brooks & Mercier, 1994, Billat *et al.*, 2003, Brun *et al.*, 2007). More recently, an interrelationship between CHO and BLC has been developed (Alkhatib, & Beneke 2008, Beneke *et al.* 2009).

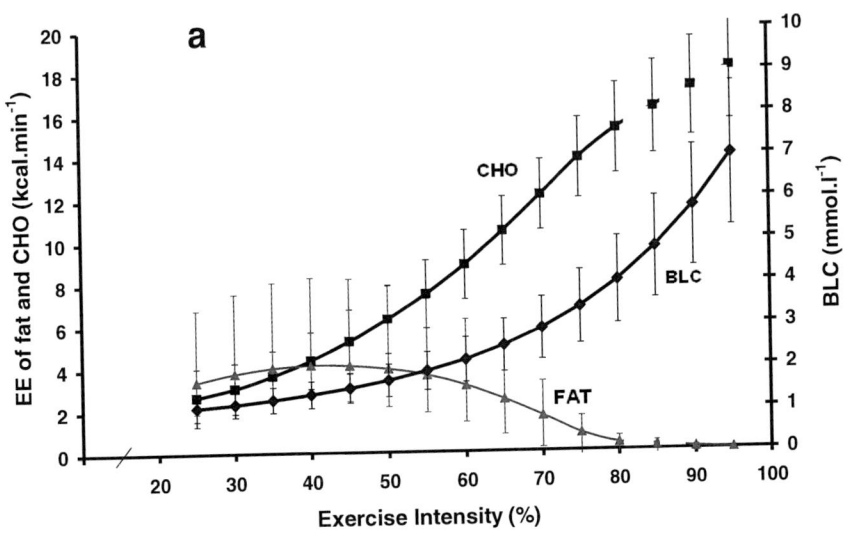

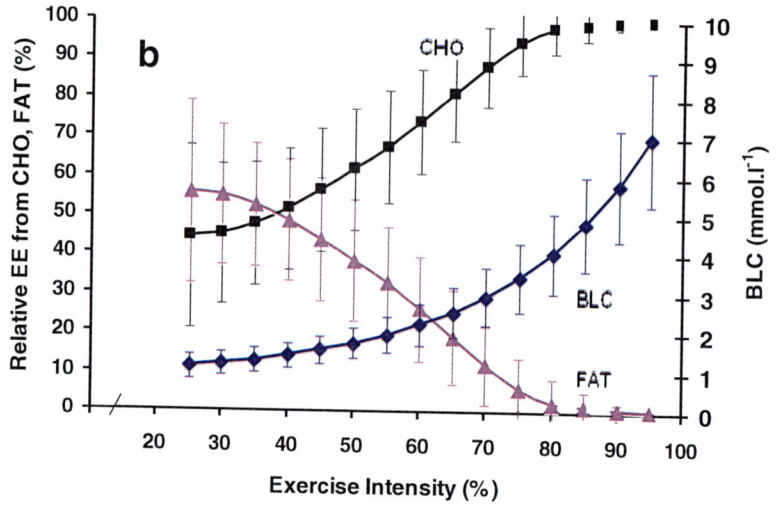

Figure 1a, 1b. The cross-over point between relative (a) and absolute (b) energy expenditure of CHO (■), and fat (▲).

AN INTERRELATIONSHIP BETWEEN LACTATE AND CARBOHYDRATE UTILISATION

Indirect calorimetry has been shown to be a valid and reliable tool to measure metabolic responses (Jeukendrup, & Wallis, 2005). It has been validated for estimation of fat and CHO oxidation for any exercise intensity up to 85% VO_{2peak} (Romijn et al., 1993). On the other hand, lactate has also been described as a metabolic substrate at different cell compartments, and was directly related to pyruvate (Wasserman et al., 1985, Henderson et al., 2004). Estimating carbohydrates and fat metabolism using indirect calorimetry has often been described separately but in association with lactate measures (Coyle et al., 1988). However, attempts to link these substrate indicators have always lacked a complementary tool to combine the two measures of lactate and respiratory exchange ratio (RER).

A interrelationship between relative rate of carbohydrate utilisation (relCHO) and BLC has previously been suggested based on theoretical modelling and employed sigmoid approximations to describe the behaviour of many metabolic systems including the relationship between lactate and pyruvate utilisation with respect to the availability of pyruvate and oxygen (Beneke, 2003). More recently (Alkhatib, & Beneke, 2008a; Beneke *et al.*, 2009) approximated a half maximal constant ($k$el) of relCHO for each individual describing an interrelationship between relCHO and BLC, suggesting that changes in relCHO can be reflected by BLC levels. This interrelationship is based on the idea that BLC may serve as an indicator of the substrate activation of the pyruvate dehydrogenase complex and therefore relCHO can be indicated by BLC using an activation constant Kel (Beneke *et al.*, 2009) and considers a) PDH complex activation by isosteric activators including pyruvate, CoA and NAD^+; allosteric cofactors including MG^{2+}, Ca^{2+}, and Mn^{2+} with pyruvate considered one of the most potent effectors (Spriet and Heigenhauser 2002) b) the bi-directional equilibrium between pyruvate and lactate which shifts towards a higher lactate to pyruvate ratio to maintain NAD^+ for both glycolysis and aerobic CHO at high glycolytic rate. The introduced interrelationship would describe relCHO as a sigmoid function of BLC (Beneke 2009): RPY = 100 / (1 + $k$el / BLC^2) where $k$el is the constant of half maximal carbohydrate combustion.

The activation constant Kel for the latter interrelationship describes whole body relCHO measured using indirect calorimetry and whole body BLC using capillary sampling, and therefore, may provide an explanation to the inter-individual variation at COP and Fatmax independently of exercise intensity (Alkhatib, & Beneke, 2008b, Alkhatib, & Beneke 2008c), (Figure 2a. 2b).

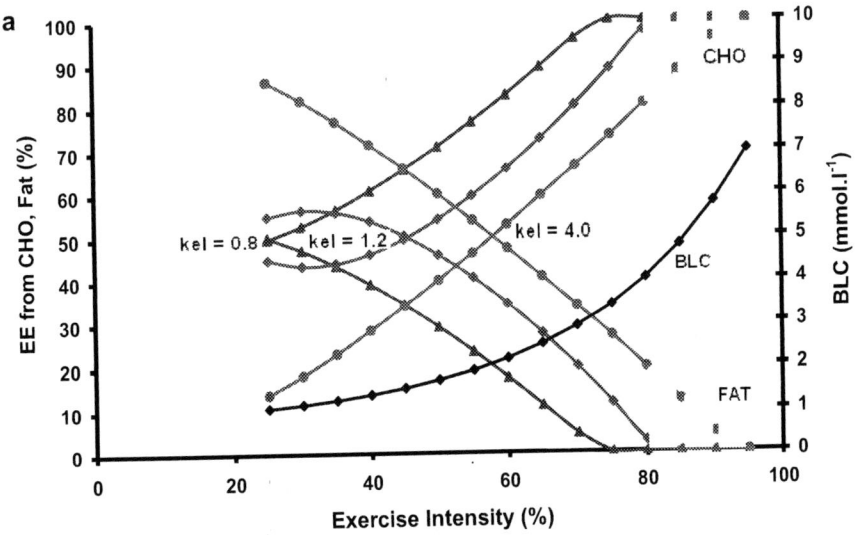

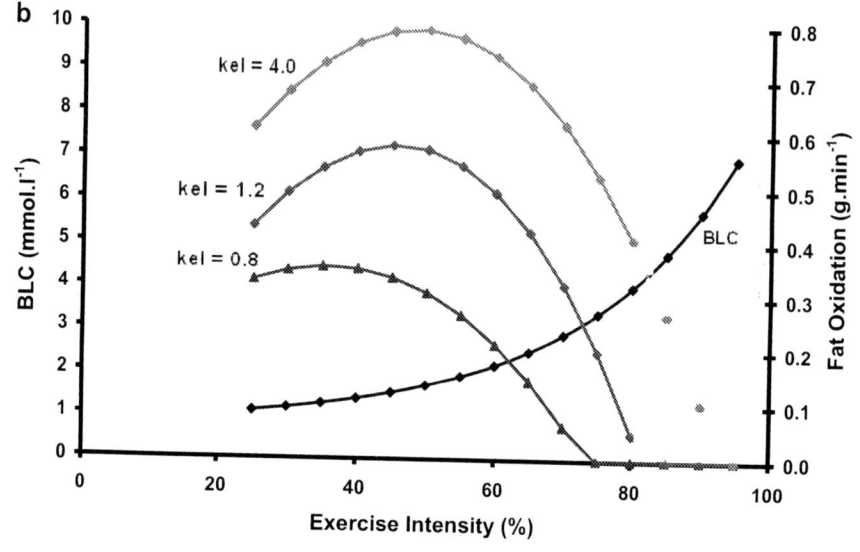

Figure 2. Example of the effects of *kel* variation on the cross-point (a) (Alkhatib, & Beneke 2008c), and the fat oxidation (b) (Alkhatib, & Beneke, 2008b). Higher *kel* induces a shift to the right in the occurrence of Fatmax, and increases the intensity difference between Fatmax and the cross-point.

There is no experimental evidence that *kel* can be changed by training. However, a potentially favourable effect for long distance performance would be a more economical use of CHO at given intensities, equivalent to an increase in *kel*, and further research in this area is recommended.

The latter proposed interrelationship may be affected by several exercise parameters such as duration (Alkhatib, & Beneke, 2009) but is independent of age and pedalling cadence (Alkhatib et al., 2005, Alkhatib, & Beneke, 2009). RER has been used extensively in recent literature to estimate indirect calorimetry for combustion of CHO and fat during exercise (Jeukendrup, & Wallis 2005). However, one must consider that indirect calorimetry assumes that the RER adequately reflects the RQ. RER reflects only the combustion of nutrient mixtures of CHO and fat and neglecting the combustion of protein. (Brooks, & Mercier 1994). Furthermore, RER is affected by the levels of VCO_2 at high exercise intensities. RER is only reliable estimate of tissue CO_2 at low exercise intensities where a stable bicarbonate pool $[HCO_3^-]$ is present. However, this is unlikely in higher exercise intensities when lactate accumulates and hydrogen ions (H^+) increase in muscles and blood. The increased H^+ will be buffered by $[HCO_3^-]$ and a non-oxidative CO_2 is exerted through hyperpnea. This causes elevated VCO_2 and therefore overestimating CHO and underestimating fat oxidation (Jeukendrup and Wallis 2005). Therefore, indirect calorimetry is only reliable when $RQ \leq 1$. During exercise, this will correspond to exercise intensities of approximately 85 % VO_{2peak} (Romijn et al., 1993). Therefore, the interrelationship between BLC and relCHO can only be characterised at submaximal exercise intensities at or below 85 % VO_{2peak} which is an essential range for exercise testing and training.

The potential practical applications of the BLC-relCHO interrelationship, and the prediction capabilities of $k$el has not been yet fully explored. There still no experimental evidence that $k$el can be changed by training. However, a potentially favourable effect for long distance performance would be a more economical use of CHO at given intensities, equivalent to an increase in $k$el, and further research in this area is recommended.

REFERENCES

Achten, J., & Jeukendrup, A. E., (2004). Relation between plasma lactate concentration and fat oxidation rates over a wide range of exercise intensities. *International Journal of Sports Medicine*, 25, 32-37.

Achten, J., Gleeson, M., & Jeukendrup, A. E., (2002). Determination of the exercise intensity that elicits maximal fat oxidation. *Medicine and Science in Sports and Exercise*, 34, 92-97.

Alkhatib, A. & Beneke, R. (2009) Effects of exercise duration on the interrelationship between lactate and carbohydrate utilisation; Abstract Book (S131); *British Association of Sport and Exercise Science Annual Conference*; Leeds Metropolitan University, Leeds UK

Alkhatib, A., & Beneke, R. (2008a). Interrelationship between lactate and carbohydrate utilisation. *European College of Sport Science*, Abstract Book (pp 519); Lisbon, Portugal

Alkhatib, A., & Beneke, R. (2008b). An interrelationship between lactate and carbohydrate utilisation explains the inter-individual variations in the cross-over point; *Journal of Sports Sciences*, (Abstract), 26(S2): S145; British Association of Sport and Exercise Science; London, UK

Alkhatib, A. & Beneke, R. (2008c). Can an interrelationship between lactate and carbohydrate utilisation explain the inter-individual variations in

Fatmax? *European College of Sport Science*, Abstract Book (pp 600-601); Lisbon, Portugal

Alkhatib, A., & Beneke, R. (2005). Description of the blood lactate concentration to incremental exercise using 2- & 3-parameter models. *European College of Sport Science*, Book of abstracts, 232.

Beaver, W. L., Wasserman, K., & Whipp, B. J. (1986). A New Method for Detecting Anaerobic Threshold by Gas-Exchange. *Journal of Applied Physiology*, 60, 2020-2027.

Bell, C., Kowalchuk, J. M., Paterson, D. H., Scheuermann, B. W., & Cunningham, D. A. (1999). The effects of caffeine on the kinetics of O-2 uptake, CO2 production and expiratory ventilation in humans during the on-transient of moderate and heavy intensity exercise. *Experimental Physiology*, 84, 761-774.

Below, P. R., Mora-Rodriguez, R., Gonzalez-Alonso, J., & Coyle, E. F. (1995). Fluid and carbohydrate ingestion independently improve performance during 1 h of intense exercise. *Medicine and Science in Sports and Exercise*, 27, 200-210.

Beneke, R, Hütler, M., & Leithäuser, R. (2009). Carbohydrate and fat metabolism related to blood lactate in boys and male adolescents; *European Journal of Applied Physiology*, 105, 257-63.

Beneke, R. (2003). Maximal lactate steady state concentration (MLSS): experimental and modelling approaches. *European Journal of Applied Physiology and Occupational Physiology*, 88, 361-369.

Beneke, R., Hutler, M. & Leithauser, R. M. (2000). Maximal lactate-steady-state independent of performance. *Medicine and Science in Sports and Exercise*, 32, 1135-1139.

Beneke, R. & vonDuvillard, S. P. (1996). Determination of maximal lactate steady state response in selected sports events. *Medicine and Science in Sports and Exercise*, 28, 241-246.

Bergman, B. C., & Brooks, G. A. (1999). Respiratory gas-exchange ratios during graded exercise in fed and fasted trained and untrained men. *Journal of Applied Physiology*, 86, 479-487.

Billat, V., Sirvent, P., Lepretre, P. M., & Koralsztein, J. P. (2004). Training effect on performance, substrate balance and blood lactate concentration at maximal lactate steady state in master endurance-runners. *Pflugers Archiv.European Journal of Physiology*, 447, 875-883.

Billat, V. L., Sirvent, P., Py, G., Koralsztein, J. P., & Mercier, J. (2003). The concept of maximal lactate steady state: a bridge between biochemistry, physiology and sport science. *Sports Medicine*, 33, 407-426.

Bircher, S., & Knechtle, B. (2004). Relationship between fat oxidation and lactate threshold in athletes and obese women and men. *Journal of Sports Science and Medicine*, 3, 174-181.

Brooks, G. A., Fahey, T. D., & Baldwin, K. M. (2005). *Exercise Physiology. Human Bioenergetics and Its Adaptations.* Boston; McGraw Hill.

Brooks, G. A. (1985). Anaerobic Threshold - Review of the Concept and Directions for Future-Research. *Medicine and Science in Sports and*

Brun, J. F., Jean, E., Ghanassia, E., Flavier, S. & Mercier, J. (2007). Metabolic training: new paradigms of exercise training for metabolic diseases with exercise calorimetry targeting individuals. *Annales de Readaptation et de Medicine Physique.*

Chambers E. S., Bridge, M. W., & Jones, D. A. (2009). Carbohydrate sensing in the human mouth: effects on exercise performance and brain activity. *Journal of Physiology*, 587,1779-94.

Coyle, E. F., Jeukendrup, A. E., Wagenmakers, A. J. M., & Saris, W. H. M. (1997). Fatty acid oxidation is directly regulated by carbohydrate metabolism during exercise. *American Journal of Physiology-Endocrinology and Metabolism*, 36, E268-E275.

Coyle, E. F., Coggan, A. R., Hopper, M. K., & Walters, T. J. (1988). Determinants of Endurance in Well-Trained Cyclists. *Journal of Applied Physiology*, 64, 2622-2630.

Dennis, S. C., Noakes, T. D., & Bosch, A. N. (1992). Ventilation and blood lactate increase exponentially during incremental exercise. *Journal of Sports Sciences*, 10, 437-449.

Gaesser, G. A., & Poole, D. C. (1996). The slow component of oxygen uptake kinetics in humans. *Exercise and Sport Science Reviews*, 24, 35-71.

Goodwin, M. L., Harris, J.E., Hernández A., & Gladden, B. L. (2007). Blood Lactate Measurements and Analysis during Exercise: A Guide for Clinicians. Journal of Diabetes Science and Technology, 1, 558–569

Gladden, L. B. (2000). The role of skeletal muscle in lactate exchange during exercise: introduction. *Medicine and Science in Sports and Exercise*, 32, 753-755.

Gollnick, P. D., Piehl, K., & Saltin, B. (1974). Selective glycogen depletion pattern in human muscle fibres after exercise of varying intensity and at varying pedalling rates. *Journal of Physiology*, 241, 45-57.

Gonzalez-Haro, C., Galilea, P. A., Gonzalez-de-Suso, J. M., Drobnic, F., & Escanero, J. F. (2007). Maximal lipidic power in high competitive level triathletes and cyclists. *British Journal of Sports Medicine*, 41, 23-28.

Jeukendrup, A. E., & Wallis, G. A. (2005). Measurement of substrate oxidation during exercise by means of gas exchange measurements. *International Journal of Sports Medicine*, 26, S28-S37.

Hargreaves, M., & Spriet, L. L. (2006). *Exercise Metabolism*; Chapter 3:PP106 - 136 Human Kinetics, USA.

Hargreaves, M. (2004). Muscle glycogen and metabolic regulation. *Proceedings of the Nutritional Society*, 63, 217-220.

Hill, A. V., Long, C. N., & Lupton, H. (1924). The effect of fatigue on the relation between work and speed, in contraction of human arm muscles. *Journal of Physiology*, 58, 334-337.

Howley, E. T., Bassett, D. R., Jr., & Welch, H. G. (1995). Criteria for maximal oxygen uptake: review and commentary. *Medicine and Science in Sports and Exercise*, 27, 1292-1301.

Henderson, G. C., Horning, M. A., Lehman, S. L., Wolfel, E. E., Bergman, B. C., & Brooks, G. A. (2004). Pyruvate shuttling during rest and exercise before and after endurance training in men. *Journal of Applied Physiology*, 97, 317-325.

Hill, A. V., Long, C. N., & Lupton, H. (1924). The effect of fatigue on the relation between work and speed, in contraction of human arm muscles. *Journal of Physiology*, 58, 334-337.

House of Commons Health Committee, The. (2004). Report on obesity (*Health - Third report (HC 23-I, Session 2003-4)*).

Hughson, R. L., Weisiger, K. H., & Swanson, G. D. (1987). Blood Lactate Concentration Increases As A Continuous Function in Progressive Exercise. *Journal of Applied Physiology*, 62, 1975-1981.

Kang, J., Hoffman, J. R., Wendell, M., Walker, H., & Hebert, M. (2004). Effect of contraction frequency on energy expenditure and substrate utilisation during upper and lower body exercise. *British Journal of Sports Medicine*, 38, 31-35.

Margaria, R., Edwards, H. T., & Dill, D. B. (1933). The possible mechanisms of contracting and paying the oxygen debt and the role of lactic acid in muscular contraction. *American Journal of Physiology*, 106, 689-715.

McGarry, J. D., Mills, S. E., Long, C. S., & Foster, D. W. (1983). Observations on the Affinity for Carnitine, and Malonyl-Coa Sensitivity, of Carnitine Palmitoyltransferase-I in Animal and Human-Tissues - Demonstration of the Presence of Malonyl-Coa in Non-Hepatic Tissues of the Rat. *Biochemical Journal*, 214, 21-28.

Ozyener, F., Rossiter, H. B., Ward, S. A., & Whipp, B. J. (2001). Influence of exercise intensify on the on- and off-transient kinetics of pulmonary oxygen uptake in humans. *Journal of Physiology-London*, 533, 891-902.

Ranallo, R. F., & Rhodes, E. C. (1998). Lipid metabolism during exercise. *Sports Medicine*, 26, 29-42.

Romijn, J. A., Coyle, E. F., Sidossis, L. S., Gastaldelli, A., Horowitz, J. F., Endert, E., & Wolfe, R. R. (1993). Regulation of endogenous fat and carbohydrate metabolism in relation to exercise intensity and duration. *American Journal of Physiology*, 265, E380-E391.

Spriet, L. L., & Heigenhauser, G. J. F. (2002). Regulation of pyruvate dehydrogenase (PDH) activity in human skeletal muscle during exercise. *Exercise and Sport Sciences Reviews*, 30, 91-95.

Spriet, L. L., Howlett, R. A., & Heigenhauser, G. J. F. (2000). An enzymatic approach to lactate production in human skeletal muscle during exercise. *Medicine and Science in Sports and Exercise*, 32, 756-763.

Starritt, E. C., Howlett, R. A., Heigenhauser, G. J. F., & Spriet, L. L. (2000). Sensitivity of CPT I to malonyl-CoA in trained and untrained human skeletal muscle. *American Journal of Physiology-Endocrinology and Metabolism*, 278, E462-E468.

Stockhausen, W., Grathwohl, D., Burklin, C., Spranz, P., & Keul, J. (1997). Stage duration and increase of work load in incremental testing on a cycle ergometer. *European Journal of Applied Physiology and Occupational Physiology*, 76, 295-301.

Stegmann, H., Kindermann, W., & Schnabel, A. (1981). Lactate kinetics and individual anaerobic threshold. *International Journal of Sports Medicine*, 2, 160-5.

Stringer, W., Wasserman, K., & Casaburi, R. (1995). The VCO2/VO2 relationship during heavy, constant work rate exercise reflects the rate of lactic acid accumulation. *European Journal of Applied Physiology and Occupational Physiology*, 72, 25-31.

van Loon, L. J. C., Greenhaff, P. L., Teodosiu, D. C., Saris, W. H. M., & Wagenmakers, A. J. M. (2001). The effects of increasing exercise intensity on muscle fuel utilisation in humans. *Journal of Physiology-London*, 536, 295-304.

Venables, M. C., Achten, J., & Jeukendrup, A. E. (2005). Determinants of fat oxidation during exercise in healthy men and women: a cross-sectional study. *Journal of Applied Physiology*, 98, 160-167.

Wasserman. K, Whipp, B. J., Koyal, S. N., & Beaver, W. L. (1973). Anaerobic Threshold and Respiratory Gas-Exchange During Exercise. *Journal of Applied Physiology*, 35, 236-243.

Wasserman, K., Beaver, W. L., & Whipp, B. J. (1990). Gas Exchange Theory and the Lactaic Acidosis (anaerobic) threshold. *Circulation*, 81, II-14-30.

Wasserman, K., Hansen, J. E., Sue, D. Y., & Whipp, B. J. (2005). *Principles of Exercise Testing and Interpretation*.

Wasserman, K., Beaver, W. L., Davis, J. A., Pu, J. Z., Heber, D., & Whipp, B. J. (1985). Lactate, Pyruvate, and Lactate-To-Pyruvate Ratio During Exercise and Recovery. *Journal of Applied Physiology*, 59, 935-940.

Whipp, B. J. (2006). Physiological Mechanisms Dissociating Pulmonary CO2 and O2 Exchange Dynamics during Exercise. *Experimental Physiology*.

Whipp, B. J. (1994). The Slow Component of O-2 Uptake Kinetics During Heavy Exercise. *Medicine and Science in Sports and Exercise*, 26, 1319-1326.

Whipp, B. J., & Ward, S. A. (1993). Pulmonary Gas-Exchange Kinetics During Exercise - Physiological Inferences of Model Order and Parameters. *Journal of Thermal Biology*, 18, 599-604.

Winder, W. W. (2001). Energy-sensing and signaling by AMP-activated protein kinase in skeletal muscle. *Journal of Applied Physiology*, 91, 1017-1028.

Xu, F., & Rhodes, E. C. (1999). Oxygen uptake kinetics during exercise. *Sports Medicine*, 27, 313-327.

Yeh, M. P., Gardner, R. M., Adams, T. D., Yanowitz, F. G. & Crapo, R. O. (1983). Anaerobic Threshold - Problems of Determination and Validation. *Journal of Applied Physiology*, 55, 1178-1186.

INDEX

A

accelerometers, 39, 49
accuracy, 59
achievement, 48
acid, 123, 169, 172, 176, 185
activation, 69, 122, 131, 158, 159, 163, 164, 176, 177, 179, 181
activity level, 36, 39, 40, 50
adaptation, 21, 63
adaptations, 78, 132, 151, 153, 154, 155, 156, 162, 163, 164, 165, 168, 169
addiction, 146, 149
adenosine, 31, 33, 34, 122
adipocyte, 122, 135
adipose, 122, 123, 133
adipose tissue, 122, 123, 133
adiposity, 123, 125, 134, 136
adjustment, 128
adolescents, 37, 38, 40, 45, 47, 48, 140, 146, 147, 149, 150, 184
ADP, 177
adults, 37, 46, 48, 125, 142, 144, 146, 147, 150
aerobic exercise, 46, 177
afternoon, 57
age, 1, 3, 9, 11, 14, 17, 19, 23, 26, 36, 38, 40, 45, 47, 49, 56, 57, 66, 72, 73, 124, 140, 154, 168, 169, 172, 182
agent, 173
agonist, 157
alcohol, 34
alcohol use, 34
alterations, 76, 156
alternative, viii, 4, 151, 153, 155, 162
amino acids, 175
amplitude, 159, 170
ankles, 74
antagonism, 32
applications, vii, 44, 163, 169, 183
arithmetic, 59
Asia, 135
assessment, 18, 49, 73, 77, 156
assignment, 126
atherogenesis, 148, 149
athletes, 18, 21, 25, 26, 34, 53, 55, 56, 63, 64, 65, 66, 67, 72, 77, 120, 131, 132, 151, 158, 159, 161, 163, 164, 168, 174, 185
attitudes, 37
Australia, 50, 72, 74
authors, 26, 31, 32, 48, 63, 128, 143, 154, 155
availability, 129, 131, 132, 176, 177, 178, 181
awareness, 36, 47, 50

B

background, vii, 119, 121
beliefs, 6, 50

Index

beneficial effect, 24, 148
bicarbonate, 171, 182
biochemistry, 184
biomechanics, viii
blood, 9, 12, 25, 124, 126, 129, 130, 155, 168, 170, 171, 173, 174, 178, 182, 184, 185
blood pressure, 124
blood stream, 130
BMI, 40, 56, 57, 64, 146
body composition, 17, 120, 125, 128, 130, 131, 132
body density, 21
body fat, 17, 18, 19, 20, 128
body size, 69, 125
body weight, 50, 120, 121, 123, 124, 125, 131, 132, 135, 136, 145
bone, 122, 130
bone resorption, 122
boredom, 147
boys, 35, 37, 39, 40, 41, 42, 43, 44, 142, 143, 144, 148, 184
brain, 31, 173, 179, 185
brain activity, 185

C

caffeine, vii, 1, 2, 3, 4, 5, 6, 7, 23, 24, 25, 26, 27, 28, 30, 31, 32, 33, 34, 184
calcitonin, 135
calcium, viii, 119, 120, 121, 122, 123, 124, 125, 126, 127, 128, 130, 131, 132, 133, 134, 135, 136, 137
caloric restriction, 124, 128
calorie, 126, 128
calorimetry, 143, 180, 181, 182, 185
cancer, 148
capillary, 12, 171, 181
carbohydrate, viii, 6, 33, 168, 169, 176, 179, 180, 183, 184, 185, 187
carbohydrate metabolism, 179, 185, 187
carbohydrates, 169, 180
carbon, 170
carbon dioxide, 170
cardiac output, 171

cardiovascular disease, 48, 172
cardiovascular function, 32
cell, 173, 180
central nervous system, 26, 31
children, vii, 36, 37, 46, 50, 51, 125, 140, 142, 144, 146, 148, 149, 150
cholecalciferol, 121, 126
cholesterol, 123
chronic diseases, 148
classes, 35, 36, 37, 39, 40, 44, 47, 48
clusters, 160, 161
CNS, 31
CO_2, 182, 184, 188
coaches, viii, 21, 26, 55, 72, 77
coefficient of variation, 59
cohort, 124
collisions, 21
combined effect, 73
combustion, 181, 182
communication, vii
community, 49, 140, 148
compensation, 171
competitive sport, 3
competitors, 64, 70
components, 30, 170
composition, 120, 123, 131, 132
computer use, 150
concentration, 27, 127, 128, 168, 171, 172, 174, 177, 183, 184
conditioning, vii, 18, 21, 27, 39, 46, 47, 48, 49, 71, 72, 77, 152, 162, 163
confidence, 67, 68
confidence interval, 67, 68
conflict, 30, 156
consensus, 49, 147
constant load, 167, 172, 174
consumers, 141
consumption, 1, 3, 24, 26, 30, 31, 32, 171
contact time, 161, 163
control, 1, 3, 4, 23, 26, 27, 28, 31, 36, 44, 53, 55, 56, 63, 64, 65, 66, 123, 125, 128, 132, 147, 158
control condition, 2, 4, 24, 27, 28, 31
control group, 53, 63, 64, 65, 66, 128
conversion, 173

correlation, 121, 124, 128, 131, 132
correlations, 128
cortex, 179
costs, 15
counsel, 39
coupling, 178
cross-sectional study, 187
culture, 36
curriculum, 51
cycling, 6, 7, 24, 33, 47, 131, 146
Czech Republic, 35, 50

D

data collection, 11
data set, 125
database, 120
debt, 173, 186
decay, 163
defence, 19
deficit, 120, 126, 128, 130, 132
degradation, 179
demographics, 119, 124
dependent variable, 61
descriptive indicators, 60
diabetes, 132, 140, 178
diet, 120, 121, 123, 124, 125, 126, 128, 131
dietary intake, 121
direct measure, 6, 139, 141
displacement, 74, 153
dissociation, 171
distribution, 172
down-regulation, 177
drawing, 144
duration, 11, 71, 131, 139, 146, 150, 156, 172, 175, 182, 183, 187

E

eating, 150
economic development, 50
elderly, 148
electromyography, 163
electrons, 173
elementary school, 51

e-mail, 50
EMG, 158
endothelial dysfunction, 148
endurance, 2, 7, 24, 26, 33, 47, 120, 130, 134, 158, 163, 164, 168, 169, 174, 175, 178, 184, 186
England, 19
environment, 10, 14, 140
enzymes, 121
equilibrium, 181
equity, 3
ergonomics, vii
estimating, 124
ethics, 1, 3, 11, 26
Europe, 53
European Union, 46
evening, 40
excitability, 157
excitation, 178
excretion, 123, 127, 134, 136
exercise performance, viii, 2, 23, 24, 26, 30, 31, 32, 33, 123, 140, 148, 167, 168, 169, 178, 185
exertion, 4, 6, 7, 9, 10, 12, 14, 15, 24, 26, 28, 31, 33
experimental condition, 3, 120, 132, 154
experimental design, 26, 30
expertise, 6
extensor, vii, 53, 55, 57, 58, 63, 65, 67, 68, 69, 155, 164

F

failure, 2, 7, 24, 33
fatigue, 10, 14, 26, 31, 33, 72, 74, 132, 152, 160, 162, 171, 173, 178, 186
fatty acids, 127, 129, 169
feedback, 35, 147, 158
feet, 57
females, 23, 26, 142, 144
fibers, 54
Finland, 12, 28
fitness, 38, 39, 47, 48, 55, 65, 125, 146, 149, 150, 170, 172
flexibility, 46, 47

flexor, 154
food intake, 121
football, 26
fuel, 174, 176, 177, 178, 187

G

gastrointestinal tract, 123
gender, 39, 41, 55, 139, 143
gender differences, 144
gene, 121, 136, 179
generation, 63, 149, 150, 169
genes, 179
Germany, 12, 19, 27, 74
girls, 35, 37, 39, 40, 41, 42, 43, 44, 51, 142, 143, 144, 147
glucose, 175, 176, 179
glycerol, 130
glycogen, 120, 130, 132, 171, 173, 175, 178, 185, 186
glycolysis, 173, 181
goals, 36, 37, 38, 48, 160, 161
government, iv
grades, 140
group activities, 37
groups, viii, 14, 21, 39, 46, 47, 49, 54, 56, 63, 64, 65, 70, 124, 130, 153, 155, 156, 171
growth, 155, 156
growth hormone, 155, 156
guidance, 11, 48
guidelines, 47, 51, 139, 140

H

hamstring, 164
health, 36, 38, 39, 45, 46, 47, 48, 49, 50, 52, 57, 67, 130, 139, 140, 141, 144, 146, 147, 148, 149, 178
health effects, 146
health services, 140
heart rate, 9, 12, 24, 25, 28, 142, 143, 146, 168
height, 11, 27, 40, 56, 57, 73, 74, 153, 161, 162

high fat, 124, 125
high quality instruction, 48
high school, 35, 40, 44, 52
hip, 57, 78, 143, 157
homeostasis, 130
Hong Kong, 69
hormonal control, 126
hormone, 121, 122, 126, 131, 133
house, 178, 187
Hunter, 149
hydrogen, 172, 182
hyperpnea, 183
hypertension, 120, 132, 136
hypertrophy, 76, 156, 162
hyperventilation, 171
hypothesis, 76, 120, 122, 125, 132, 156
hypoxia, 173

I

ideal, 120
identification, vii, 19, 120, 174
impairments, 148
implementation, 153
incidence, 140
inclusion, 158, 160
independent variable, 124
Indians, 178
indicators, 2, 54, 64, 65, 67, 180
individuality, 48
inertia, 21
infancy, 31
inferences, 30
informed consent, 1, 3, 11, 19, 26, 57, 72, 73
ingestion, 2, 7, 23, 24, 25, 27, 31, 32, 33, 34, 184
inhibition, 122, 136, 157, 161, 177
injuries, 57
injury, iv, viii, 163
insight, vii
instructors, 40
insulin, 136, 150, 178
insulin resistance, 136, 178
interaction, 14, 41, 169, 177, 178, 179

Index

interactions, 4, 28, 70, 150, 156
interrelationships, 169
interval, 152, 160, 161, 162
intervention, 35, 49, 50, 51, 52, 77, 120, 123, 124, 125, 126, 127, 128, 130, 132, 134, 150, 153, 155
ions, 172, 182
Italy, 150

J

Japan, 12, 37
joints, 157

K

kinetics, 164, 184, 185, 186, 187, 188
Krebs cycle, 176

L

labour, 66
lactic acid, 168, 171, 172, 186, 187
LDL, 123
learning, 3, 49
leisure, 14, 36, 37, 44, 140
leisure time, 36, 37, 44
leucine, 175
lifestyle, 36, 37, 38, 44, 45, 47, 48, 49, 124, 140, 178
limitation, 6, 144
line, 74
links, 74, 119, 121
lipid metabolism, 121, 125, 127, 133, 135
lipids, 133, 179
lipolysis, 119, 122, 129, 132, 136, 177
liver, 171
long distance, 182, 183
longevity, 36

M

males, 23, 26, 142, 144, 146, 148, 155
management, 70
manipulation, vii, viii, 160

market, 141
meals, 127, 135
measurement, 58, 72, 74, 132, 143, 147
measures, 4, 9, 10, 12, 19, 20, 24, 27, 28, 32, 51, 68, 72, 73, 75, 76, 120, 126, 130, 154, 167, 180
median, 42
membranes, 172
memory, 46
men, 22, 39, 68, 124, 133, 135, 154, 155, 164, 184, 185, 186, 187
messenger RNA, 34
meta-analysis, 7, 124
metabolic syndrome, 132
metabolism, 7, 32, 33, 120, 121, 122, 123, 126, 127, 129, 130, 132, 133, 134, 135, 136, 168, 169, 171, 176, 177, 180, 184, 187
methodological procedures, 55
mice, 121, 123, 135
mitochondria, 123, 177, 178
mobility, 148
model, 54, 55, 67, 69, 119, 124, 168, 172
models, 55, 120, 124, 127, 172, 184
morbidity, 48
mortality, 48
mortality rate, 48
motion, 74, 76
motivation, 149
motor neurons, 157
motor skills, 6
movement, vii, 55, 64, 77, 141, 144, 149, 152, 153, 159, 162
muscle strength, 70
muscles, 54, 55, 63, 65, 67, 68, 69, 78, 152, 157, 158, 159, 164, 171, 173, 176, 178, 182, 186
mutant, 121

N

nervous system, 33, 34, 163
neurons, 157
nucleus, 34
nutrition, vii, viii, 120

O

obesity, 121, 132, 134, 136, 140, 178, 187
objectives, 17
observations, 37, 39, 125, 126
order, 3, 4, 9, 23, 25, 26, 48, 49, 56, 59, 141, 148, 159
organism, 63
overload, 56, 72, 163, 164
overweight, 126, 133, 146, 148, 150
oxidation, 120, 126, 127, 128, 130, 132, 133, 134, 168, 169, 175, 176, 177, 179, 180, 182, 183, 185, 186, 187
oxidation rate, 128, 130, 132, 176, 183
oxygen, 10, 12, 131, 139, 141, 142, 143, 144, 145, 146, 167, 168, 170, 173, 181, 185, 186
oxygen consumption, 131

P

Pacific, 135
pacing, 27
pain, 26, 31
parameter, 143, 172, 174, 184
parameters, 31, 59, 60, 68, 131, 154, 167, 168, 172, 182
parathyroid, 133, 135
parathyroid hormone, 133, 135
perceptions, 52
performance indicator, 174
performers, vii, 14
personality, 6
phosphorylation, 122, 131
physical activity, vii, viii, 26, 35, 36, 37, 38, 39, 40, 44, 45, 46, 47, 48, 49, 50, 51, 52, 120, 125, 139, 140, 146, 147, 149, 150, 162, 169
physical education, 36, 44, 51
physical exercise, 63
physical fitness, 38, 39, 45, 48, 49, 65, 125
physical health, 40
physiology, vii, viii, 121, 184
placebo, vii, 1, 2, 3, 4, 5, 6, 7, 23, 24, 25, 26, 27, 28, 30, 31, 32, 34

plasma, 25, 27, 127, 131, 175, 176, 183
poor, 121
population, viii, 54, 56, 57, 63, 64, 65, 66, 67, 119, 124, 130, 147, 155, 162
Portugal, 183, 184
positive correlation, 127
positive relation, 119
positive relationship, 119
power, viii, 2, 15, 24, 25, 33, 49, 51, 53, 63, 64, 66, 70, 71, 72, 74, 75, 76, 77, 78, 129, 151, 152, 154, 161, 162, 163, 164, 165, 168, 169, 170, 179, 185
power relations, 78
prediction, 167, 183
predictors, viii, 125, 127, 168, 169
pressure, 134
prevention, 178
primary school, 40
producers, 141
production, 69, 70, 72, 75, 152, 155, 158, 170, 176, 184, 187
program, 39, 48, 153, 162, 163
proteins, 133
protocol, 1, 3, 6, 11, 130, 153, 170
protons, 173
psychology, vii, viii
public health, 38, 150
pupil, 48

Q

quadriceps, 164
quality of life, 49, 50

R

race, 27
radar, 129
range, viii, 2, 25, 27, 74, 76, 77, 119, 159, 167, 172, 183
ratings, 7, 24, 31, 33
reality, 164
reason, 125, 129, 150
receptors, 31, 34
recovery, 155, 156

Index

reflexes, 157
regeneration, 175
regression, 127, 171
regression line, 171
regulation, 122, 124, 126, 135, 186
rehabilitation, viii
relationship, 6, 119, 120, 124, 125, 126, 159, 163, 165, 170, 180, 187
relationships, 124
relaxation, 69
reliability, 50, 68
repetitions, 2, 24, 33, 72, 73, 155, 160, 161
resistance, viii, 2, 5, 7, 24, 32, 33, 68, 71, 72, 74, 76, 77, 78, 151, 153, 154, 155, 156, 163, 164, 165
resources, 168
respiratory, 127, 128, 130, 167, 168, 170, 171, 174, 180
responsiveness, 6
rewards, 38, 47
risk, 50, 141, 148, 149, 150, 178
risk factors, 141, 148, 150
RNA, 133
routines, 38
rugby, 26

S

sample, 12, 25, 53, 56, 57, 66, 67, 76
sampling, 74, 145, 181
saturated fat, 123, 133
Scandinavia, 69, 163
school, 37, 39, 40, 42, 44, 48, 49, 50, 51, 52, 150
scientific knowledge, vii
scores, 2, 4, 5, 21, 28, 31
searching, 6, 36, 141
secretion, 122
sedentary lifestyle, 37
selecting, 10
self-observation, 38
sensing, 141, 179, 185, 188
sensitivity, 65
Serbia, 53, 57, 69
serum, 122, 126, 127, 128, 133
shape, 158
shaping, 48
shortage, 121
side effects, 126
similarity, 144
skeletal muscle, 31, 54, 68, 123, 134, 156, 173, 174, 178, 185, 187, 188
skills, 1, 3, 48, 49
Slovakia, 79
software, 58, 59
Spain, 49
specificity, 65, 162
speculation, 148
speed, 11, 21, 56, 68, 145, 153, 158, 159, 162, 186
spindle, 157
sports, viii, 1, 3, 18, 21, 25, 26, 30, 32, 33, 50, 54, 64, 65, 120, 140, 184
SPSS, 4, 12, 20, 28, 40, 59, 75
stability, 10, 14, 165
stages, 25, 153
standard deviation, 59
standardization, 69
standards, 49
starvation, 175
statistics, 59, 60
stimulus, 72
storage, 122, 157, 175
strain, 6
strategies, 163
strength, vii, viii, 18, 21, 26, 46, 54, 56, 63, 68, 69, 70, 71, 72, 76, 77, 78, 151, 152, 154, 155, 156, 160, 162, 163, 164, 165
stress, 6, 10, 14, 15, 33
stretching, 158
striatum, 179
students, 40, 44, 48, 52, 57, 66, 68, 72, 73
substance abuse, 34
substrates, 120, 132, 169, 174
supervision, 48
supply, 173, 175
suppression, 123, 127, 128
surface area, 21
symptoms, 6

T

Taiwan, 149
talent, vii, 19
targeting individuals, 185
teachers, 48
teenagers, 36, 37, 44, 46, 149
television, 143, 150
TEM, 126
temperature, 123
tendon, 157, 158, 164
tension, 157, 159
testosterone, 155, 156
therapy, viii
thinking, 65
thresholds, 156, 167, 169
thyroid, 121
time commitment, 156
time periods, 54, 120, 145
tissue, 182
total cholesterol, 123
total energy, 120, 131, 132
training programs, 152, 154, 162
transcription, 179
transition, 158, 161, 167
translation, 50
transmission, 31
transport, 37, 50, 172
trial, 2, 3, 6, 25, 27, 33, 51, 58, 63, 123, 130, 131
tricarboxylic acid, 173
tricarboxylic acid cycle, 173
triglycerides, 175
turnover, 175

U

uncertainty, 121
United Kingdom, 1, 9, 17, 23, 49, 71, 119, 139, 140, 151
United States, 124, 134
university students, 50, 69
US Department of Health and Human Services, 46

V

validation, 66
validity, 10, 14, 50, 68, 76, 145
values, 12, 13, 24, 25, 28, 31, 63, 64, 65, 66, 143, 144, 145, 147, 154, 172
variability, 169
variables, 2, 12, 17, 19, 21, 28, 30, 61, 65, 66, 67, 70, 73
variance, 4, 28
variation, 27, 143, 145, 147, 162, 163, 181, 182
velocity, 18, 71, 72, 152, 153, 158, 159, 161, 163, 165, 174
ventilation, 184
venue, 47
video games, viii, 139, 141, 143, 146, 148, 149
vitamin D, 135
volleyball, 22, 70

W

walking, vii, 9, 10, 11, 12, 14, 15, 36, 37, 38, 39, 43, 44, 47, 144, 145, 150
weight changes, 123
weight gain, 121, 124, 135, 178
weight loss, 124, 126
weight management, 137, 141
wellness, 49
women, 22, 69, 125, 126, 127, 133, 164, 185, 187
work study, 132
workers, 123
workload, 128, 170, 172, 174

Y

yield, 156
young adults, 50, 147
young men, 149
young women, 133, 164